MAGICAL MANDALAS

Control Yourself With Best Alternative Meditation, Coloring Books For Adults

Mandala Craft Art

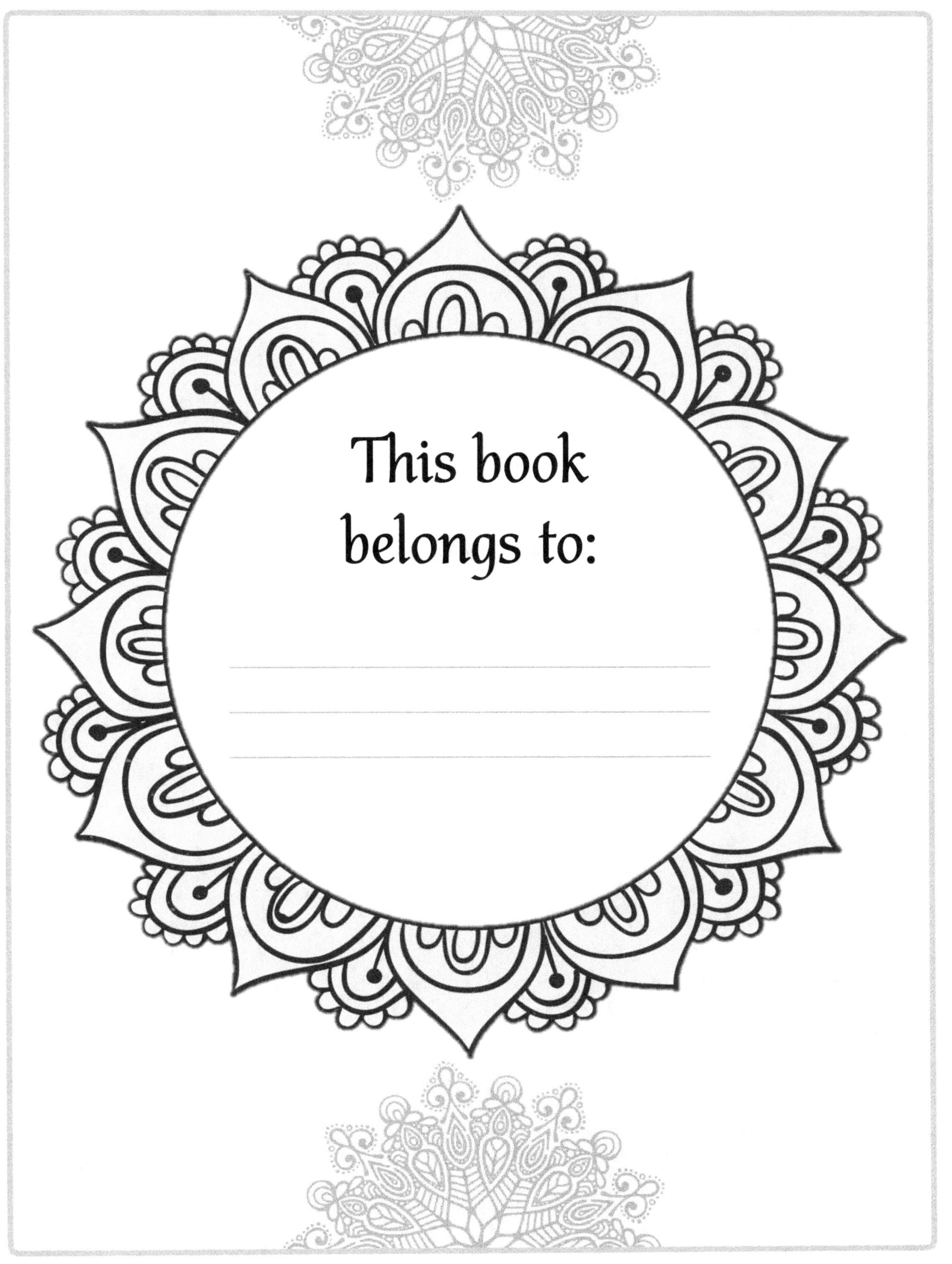
This book
belongs to:

Color Swatch

Test your color supplies on this page to see how they react to the paper. Place a blank page or two behind each page as your color, to prevent bleed-through to the next page.

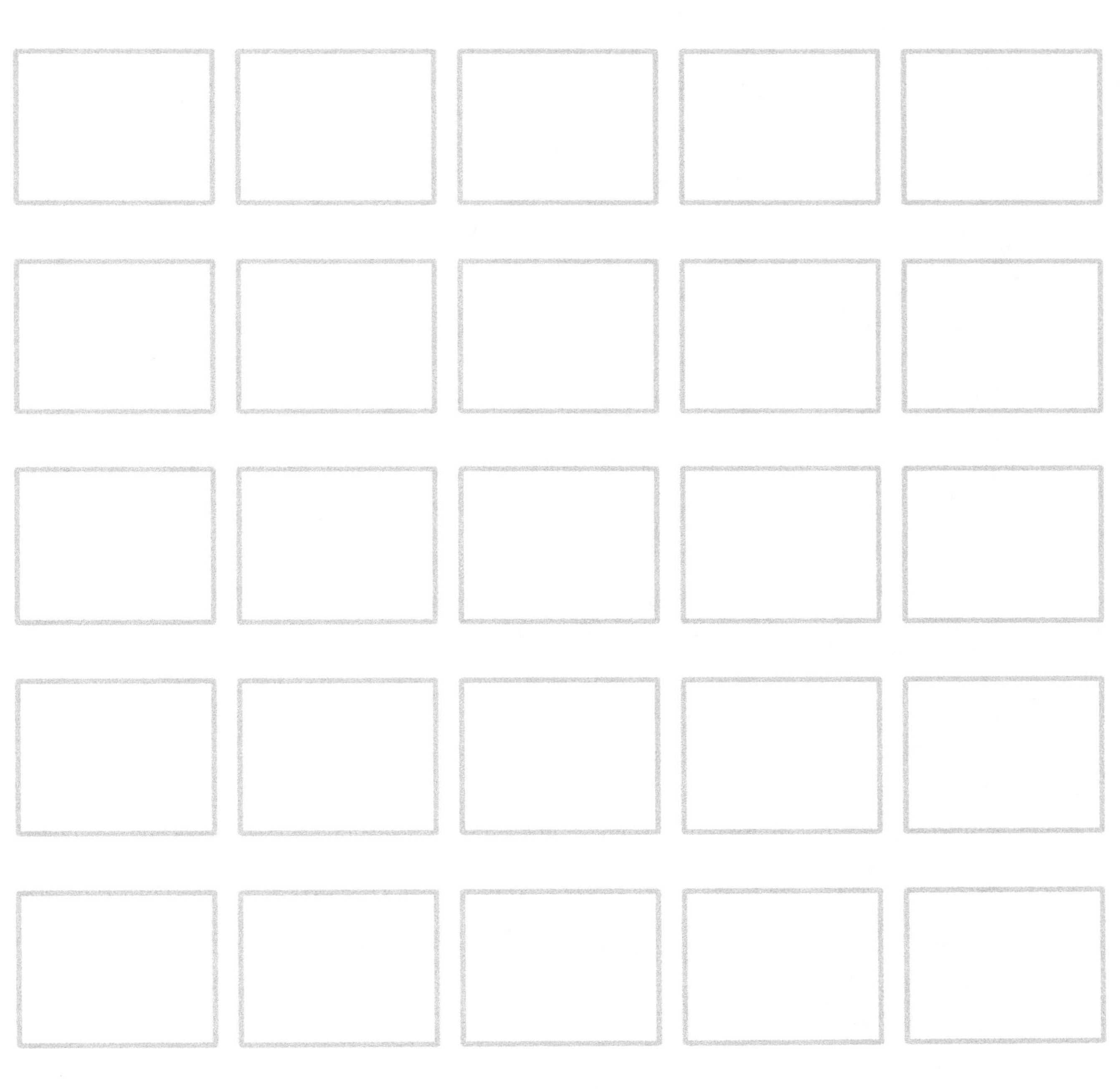

Color this mandala!

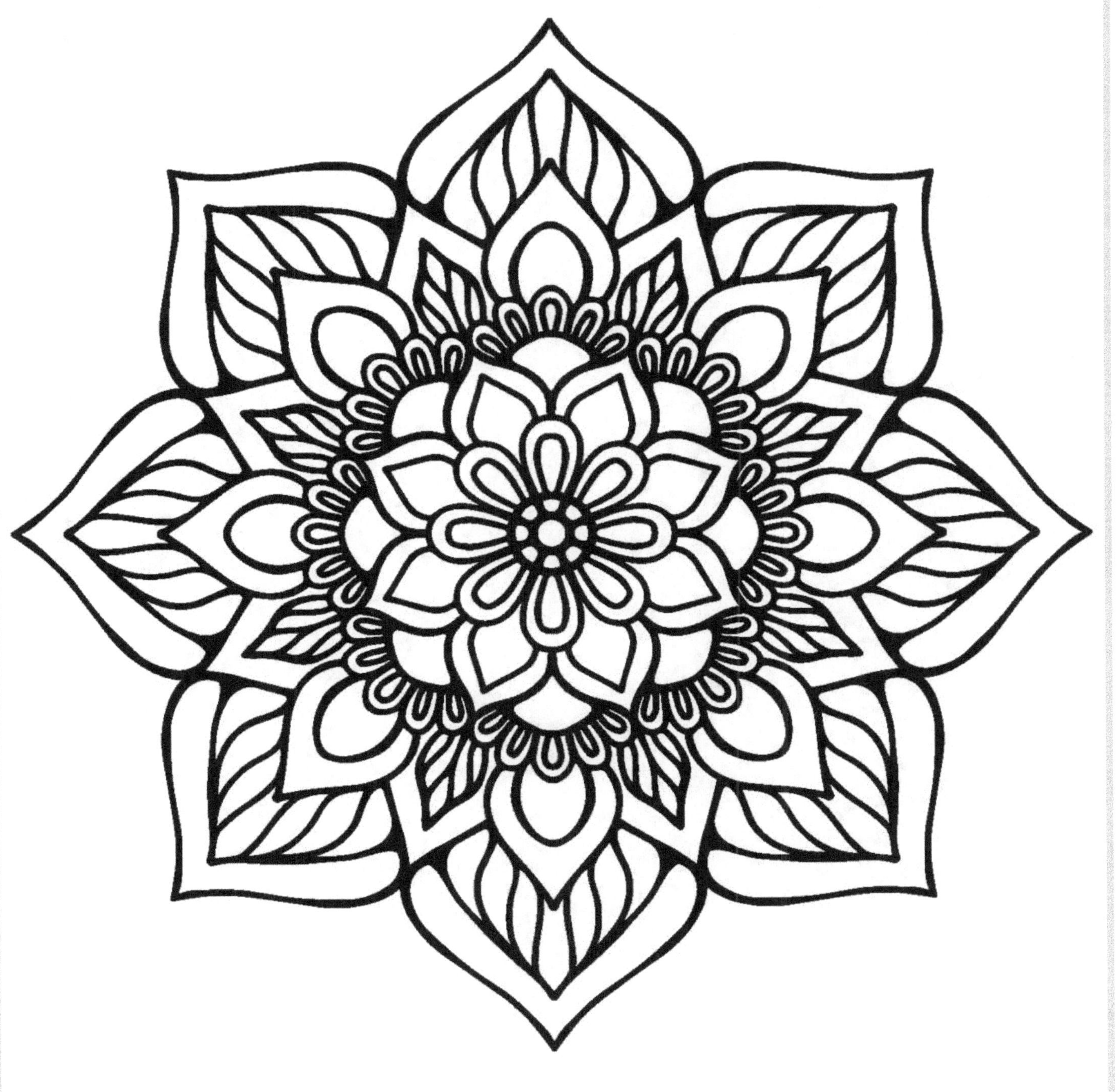

Color this mandala!

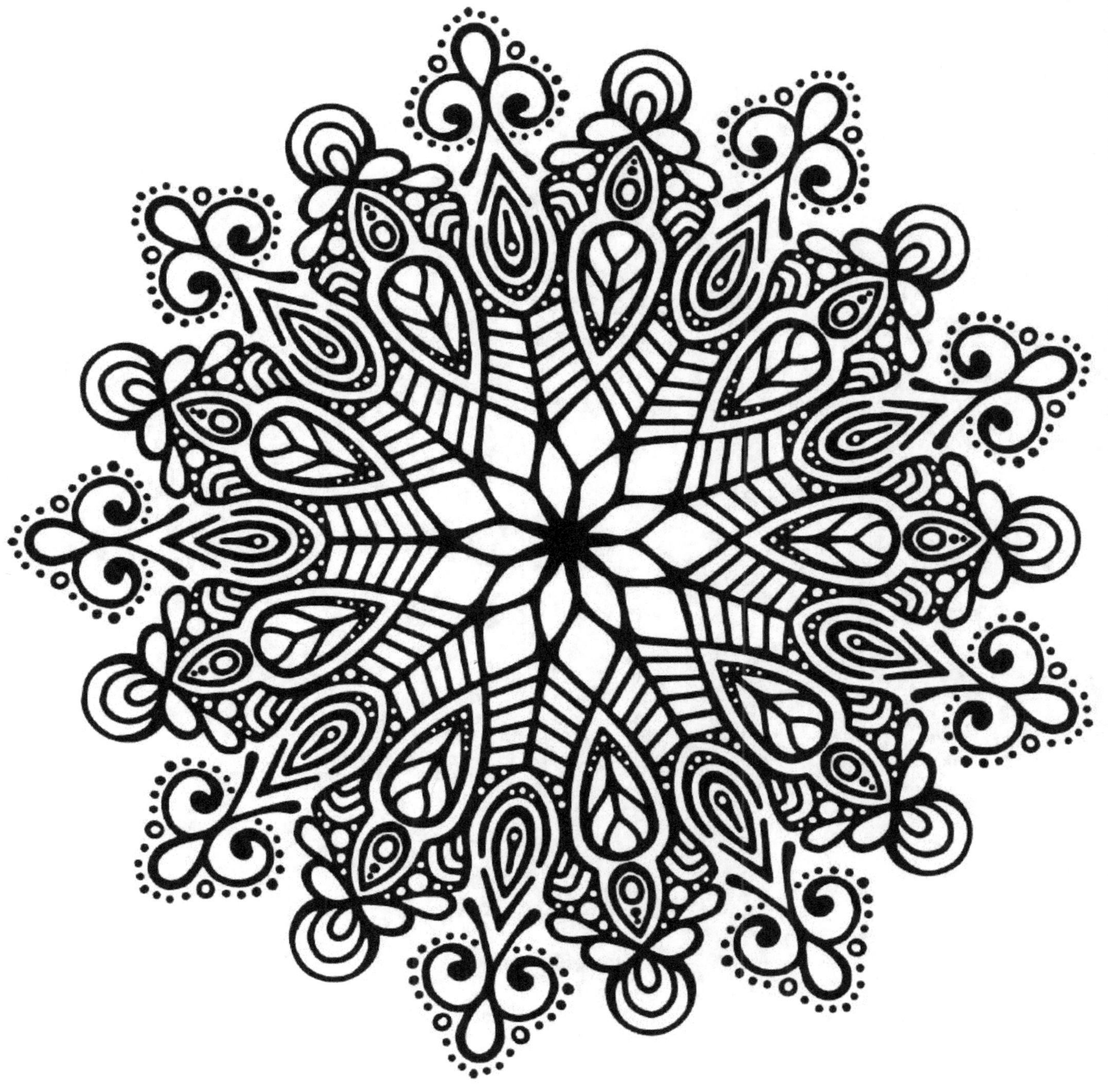

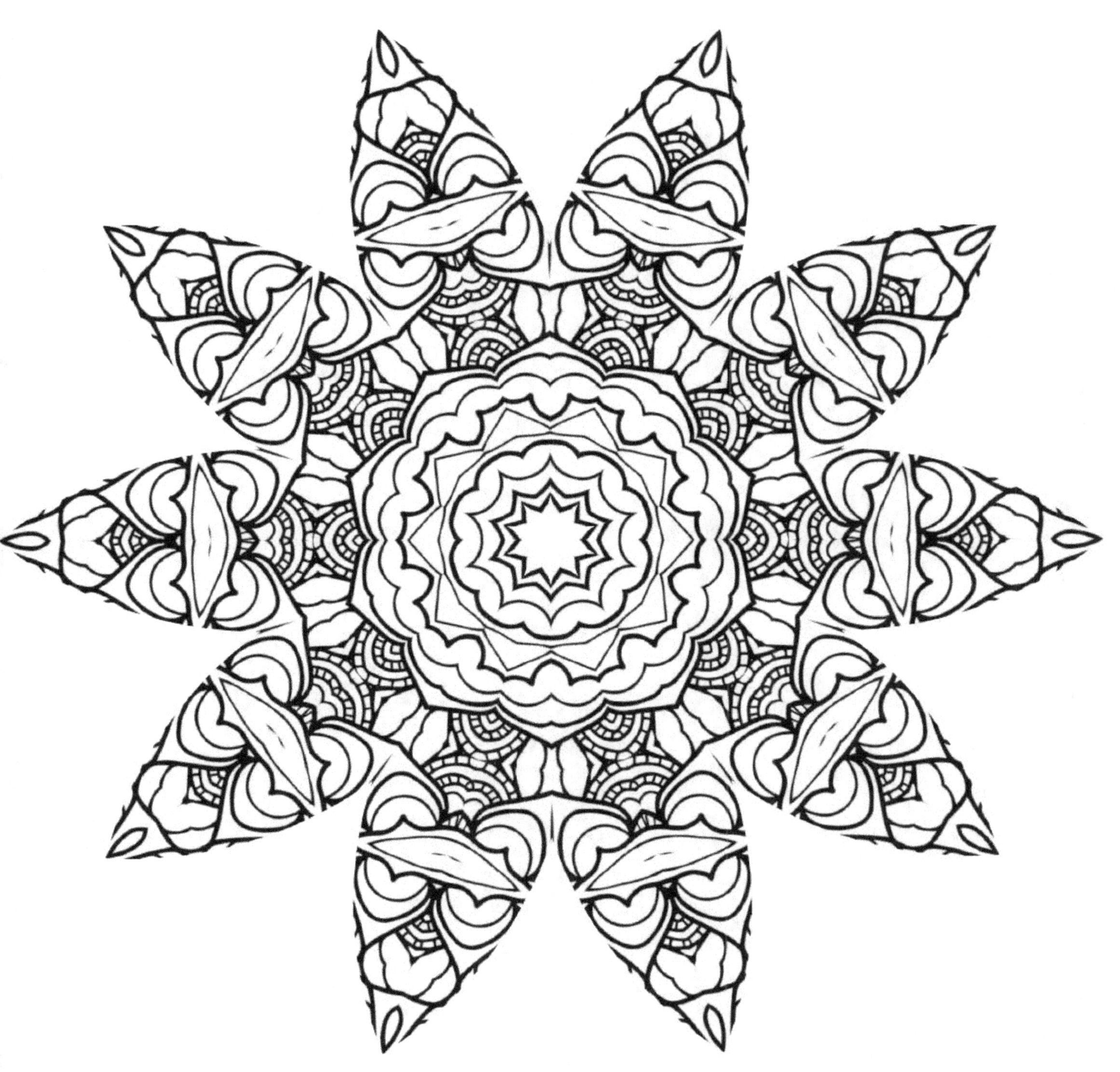

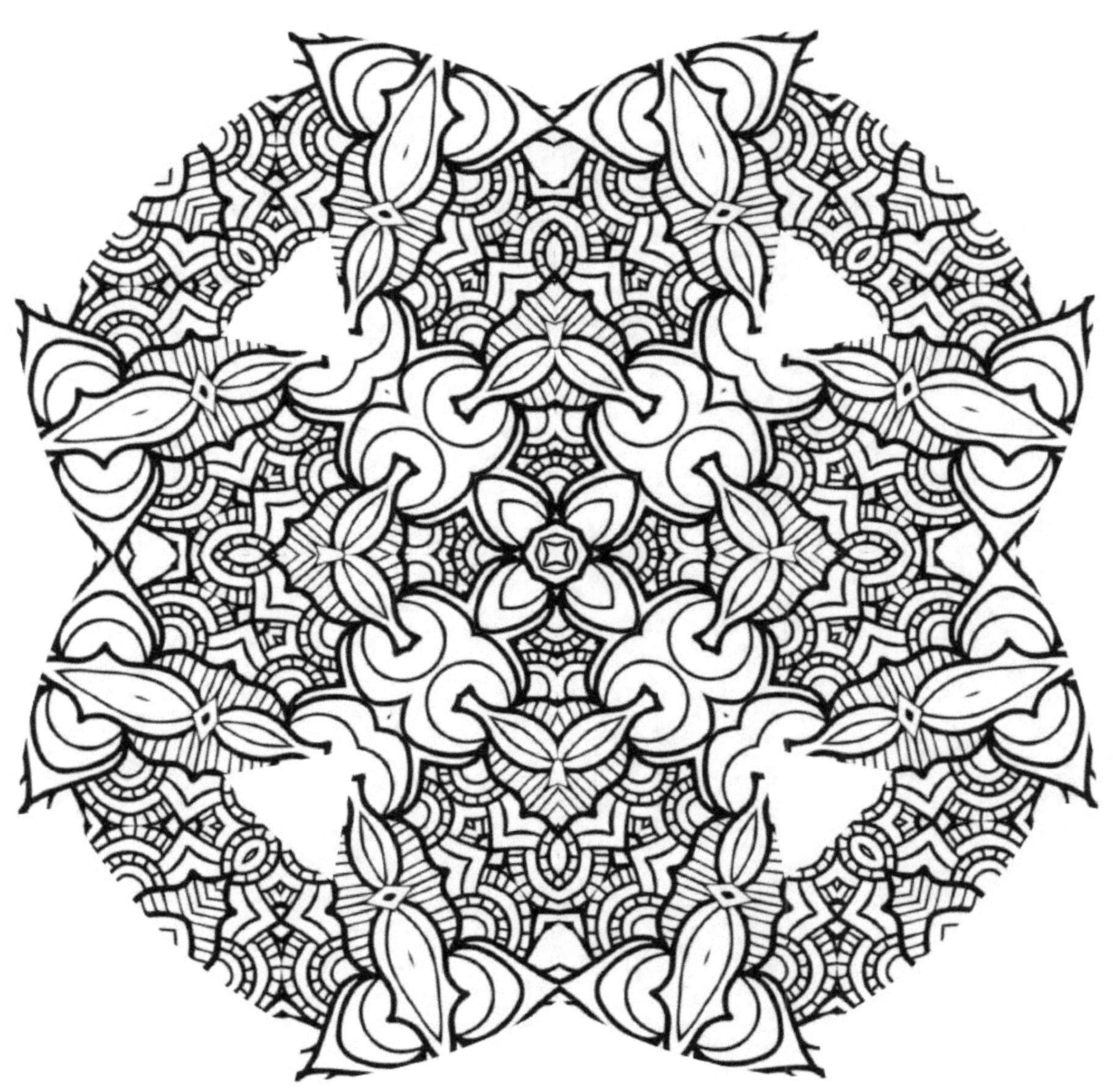

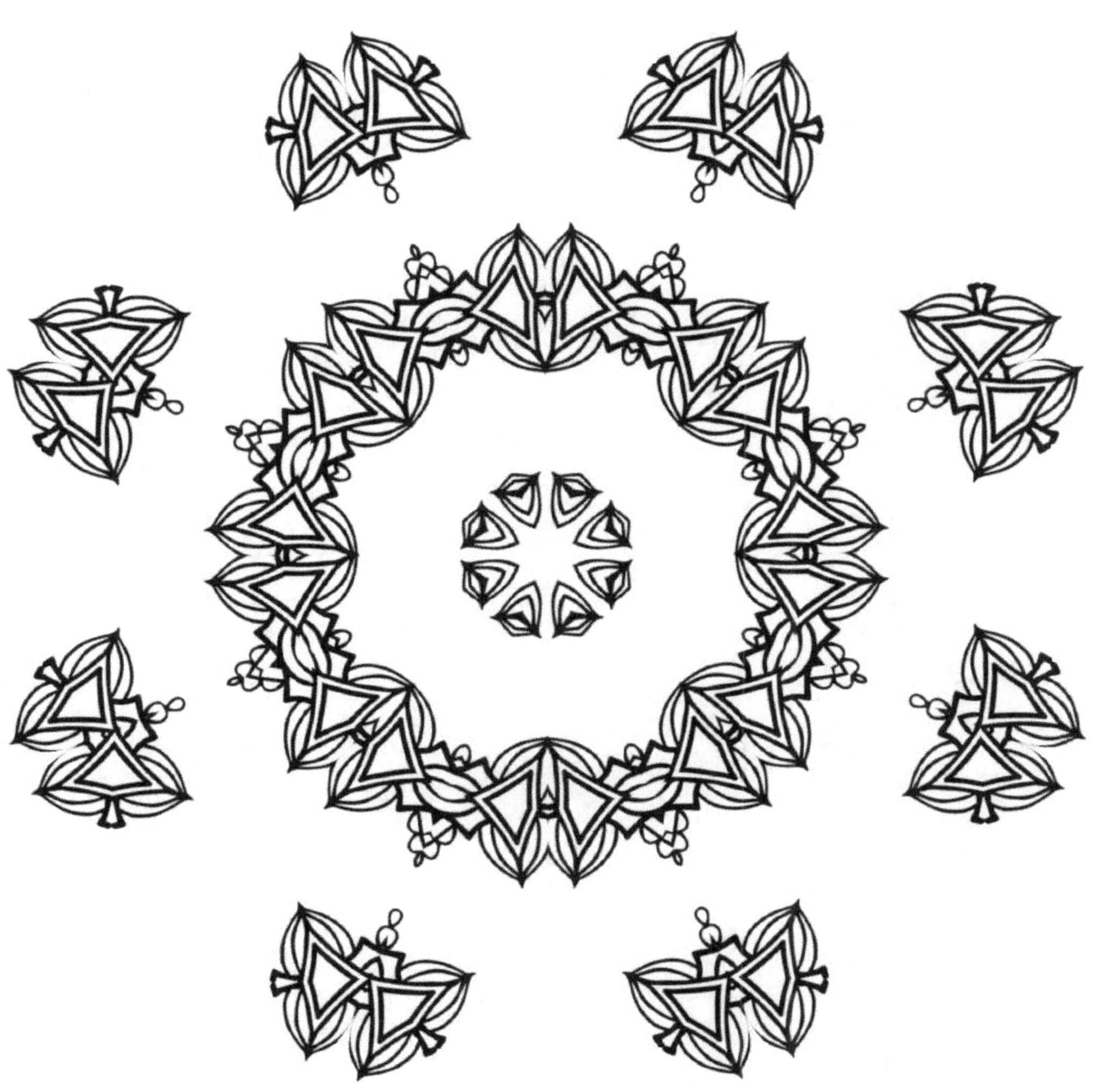

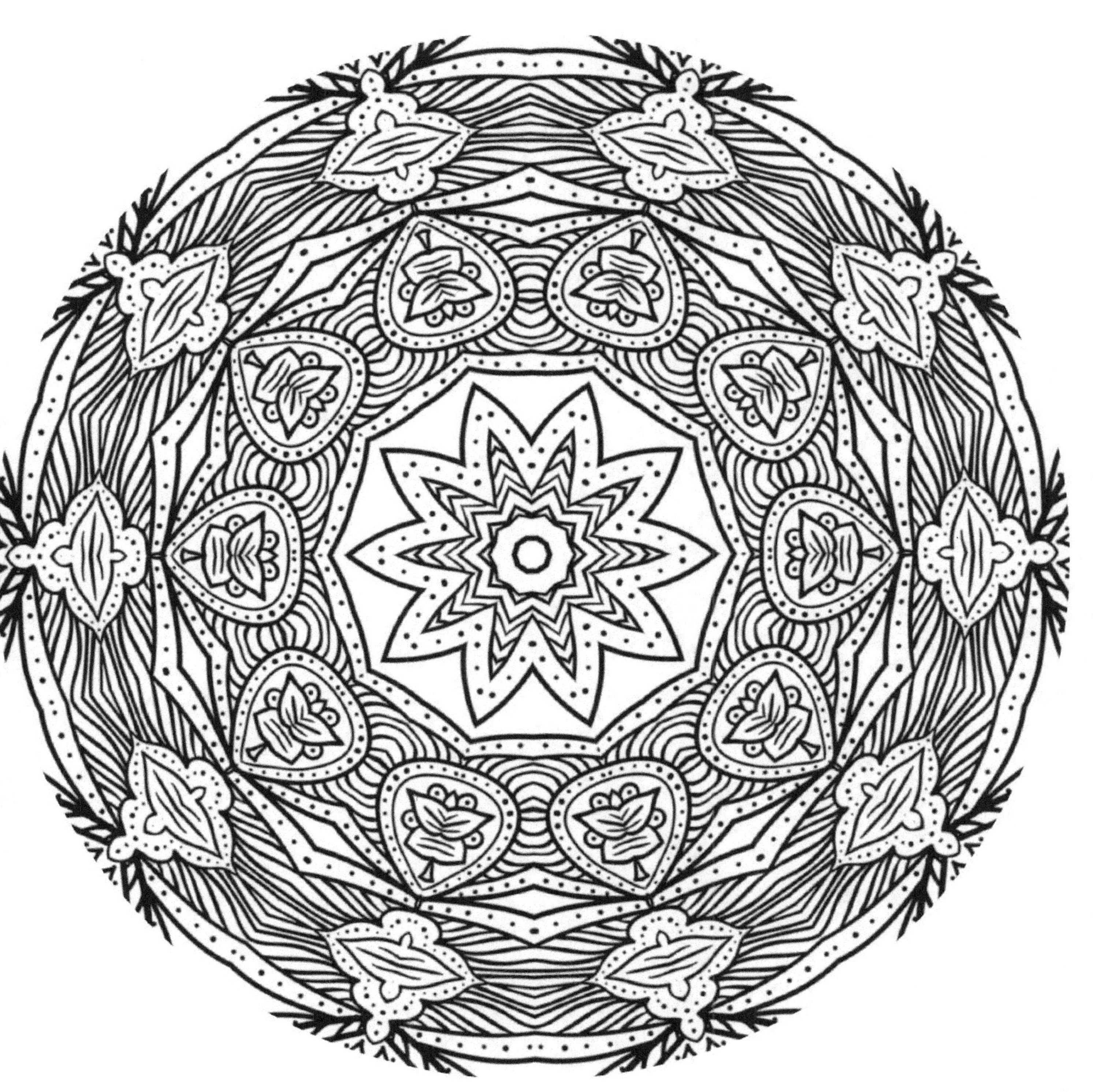

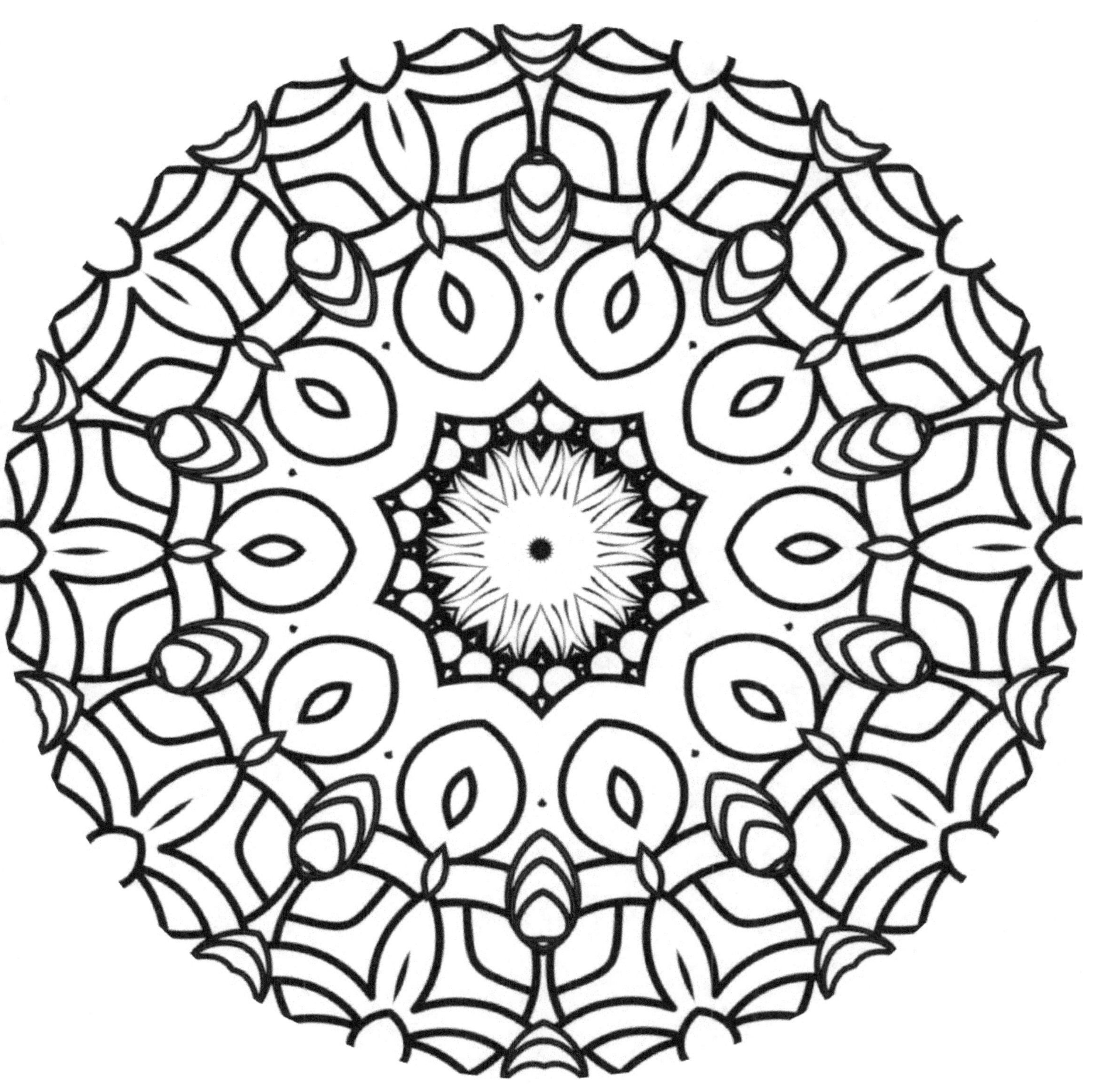

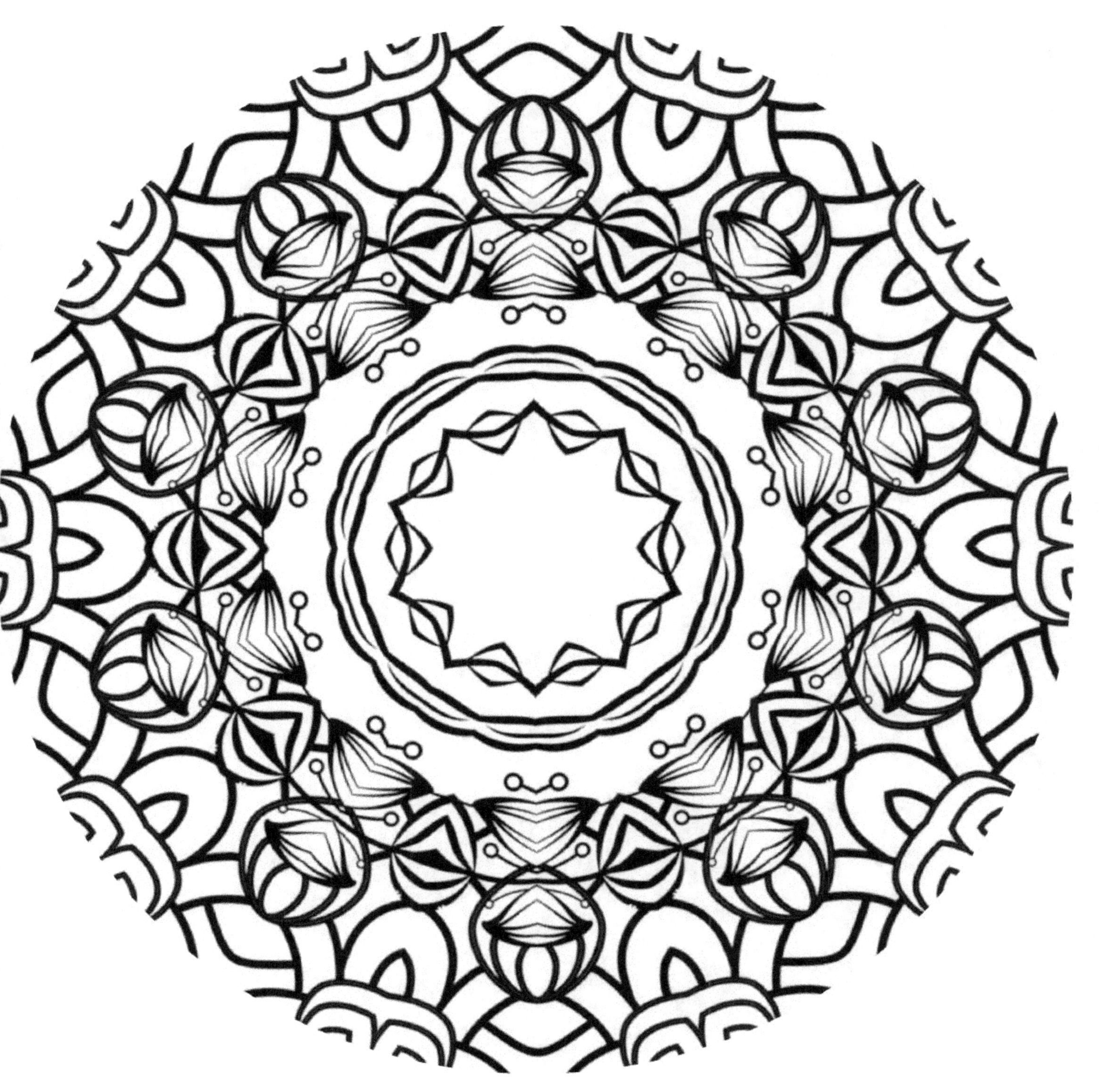

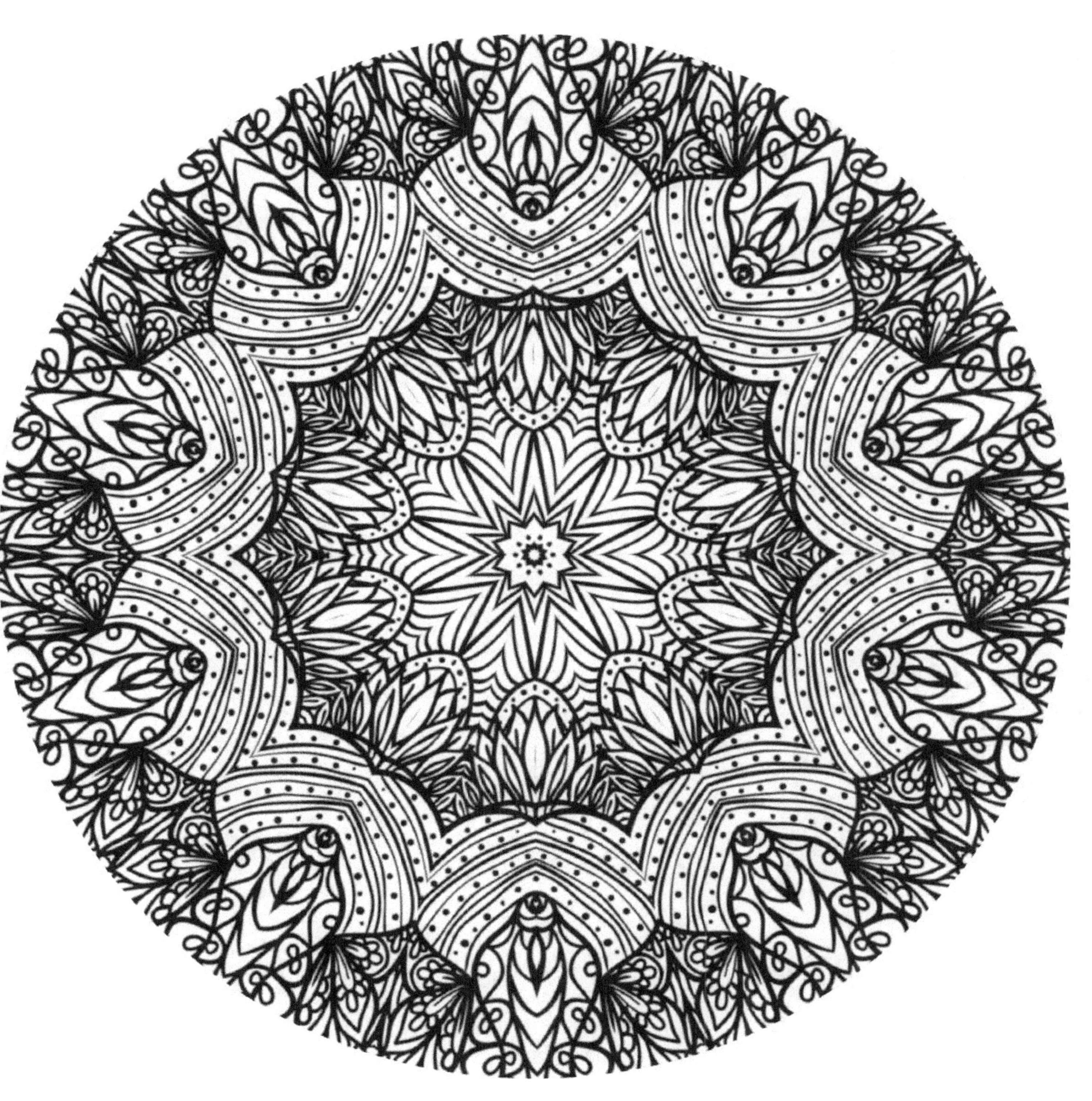

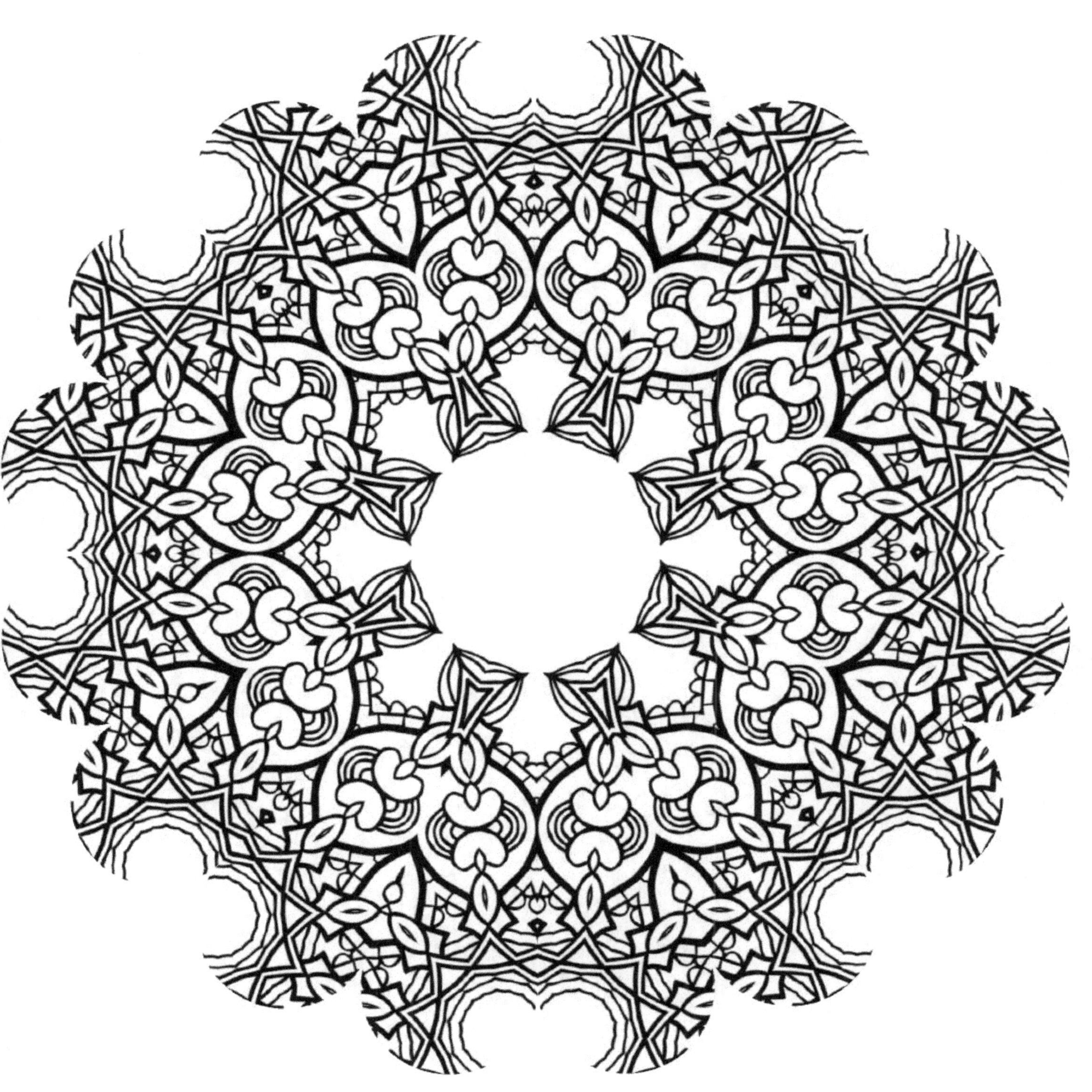

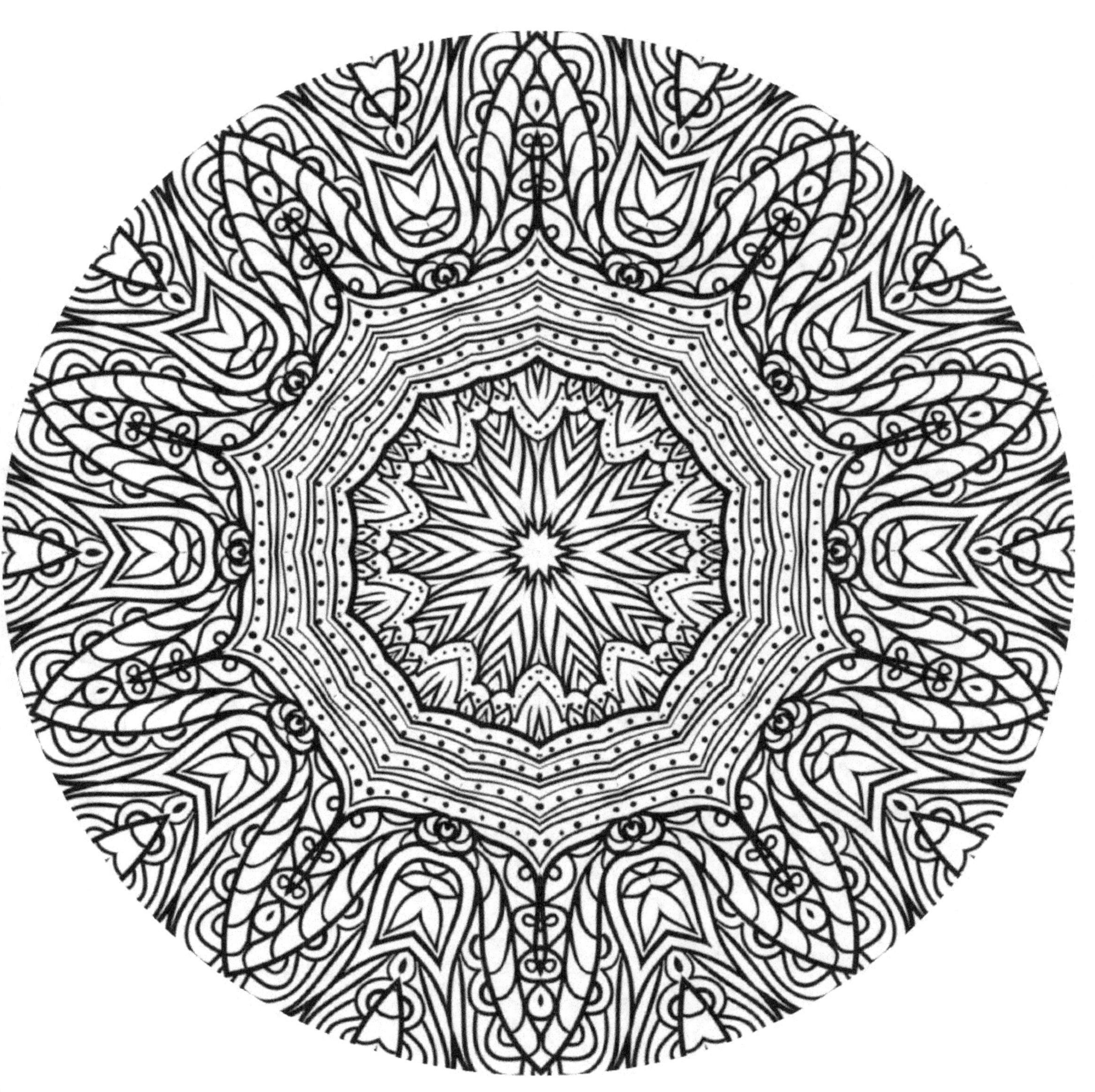

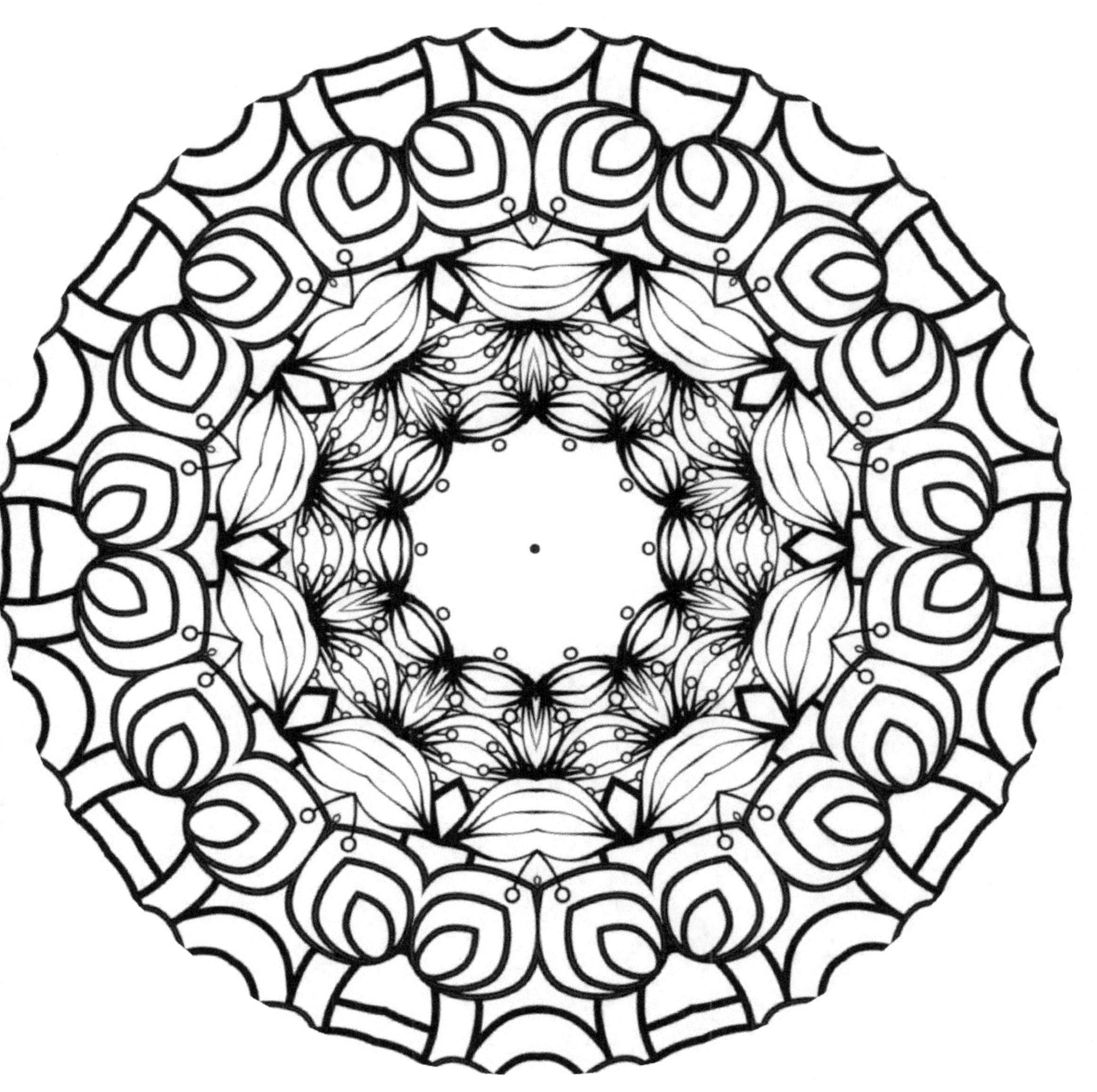

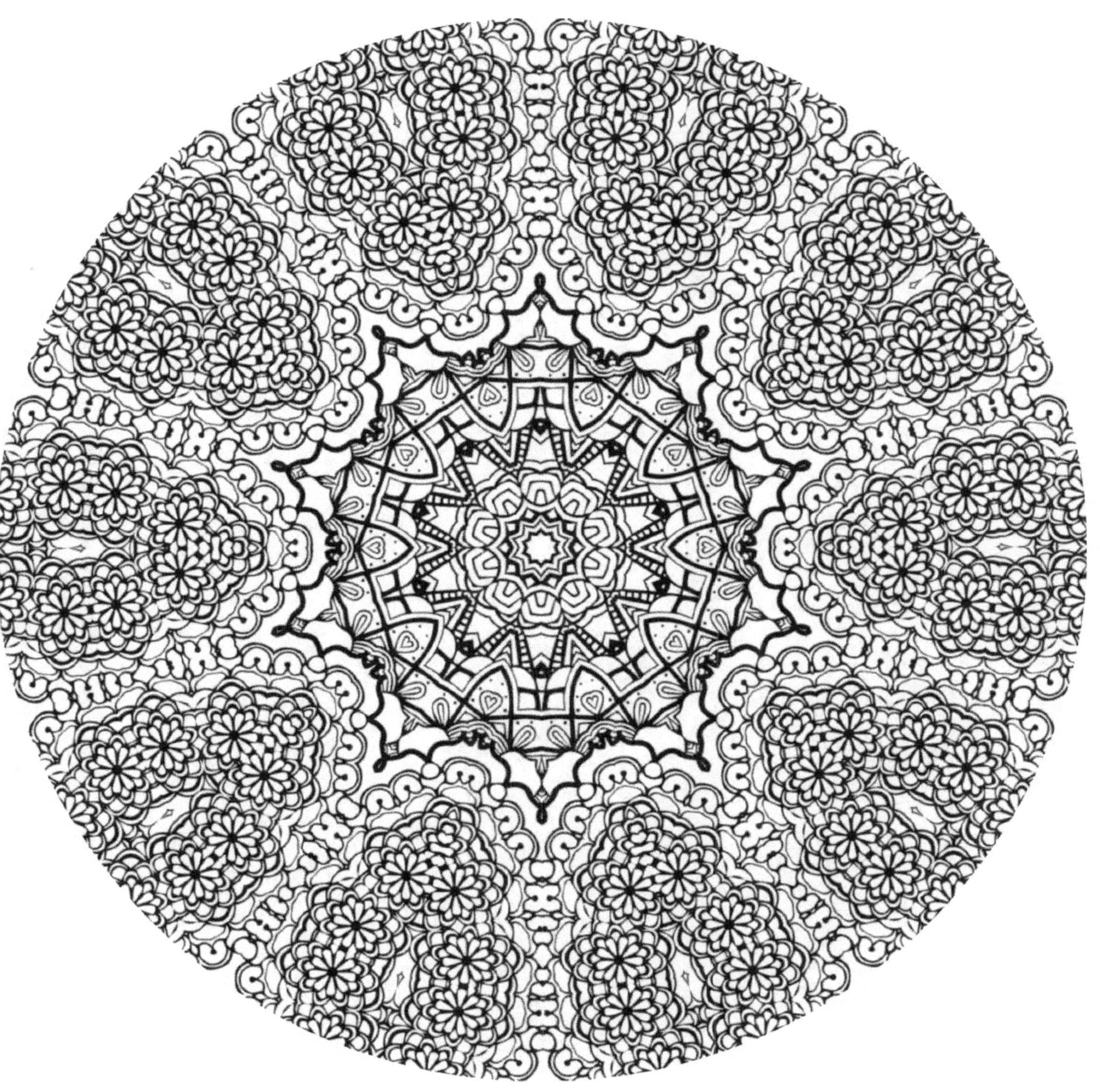

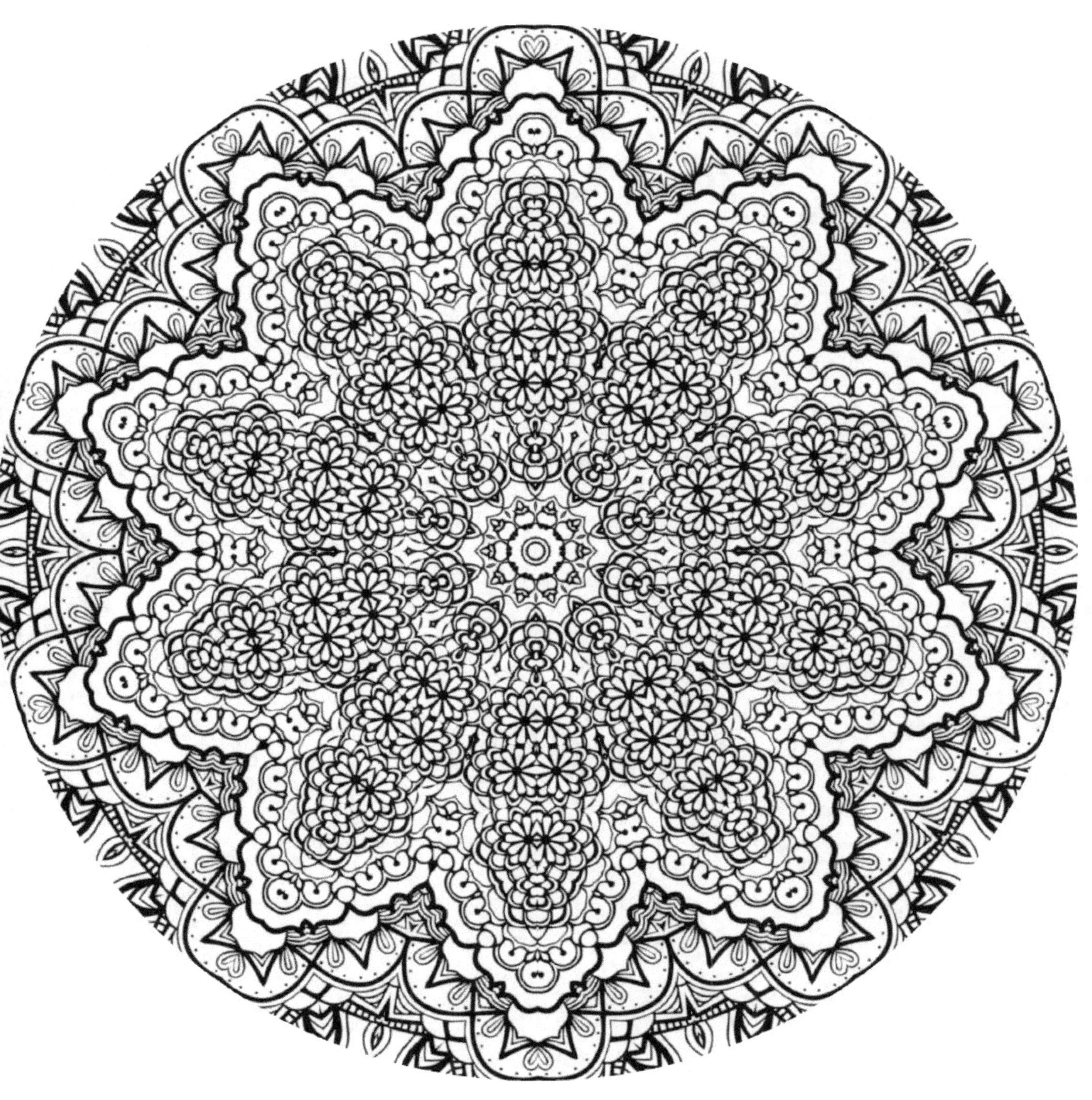

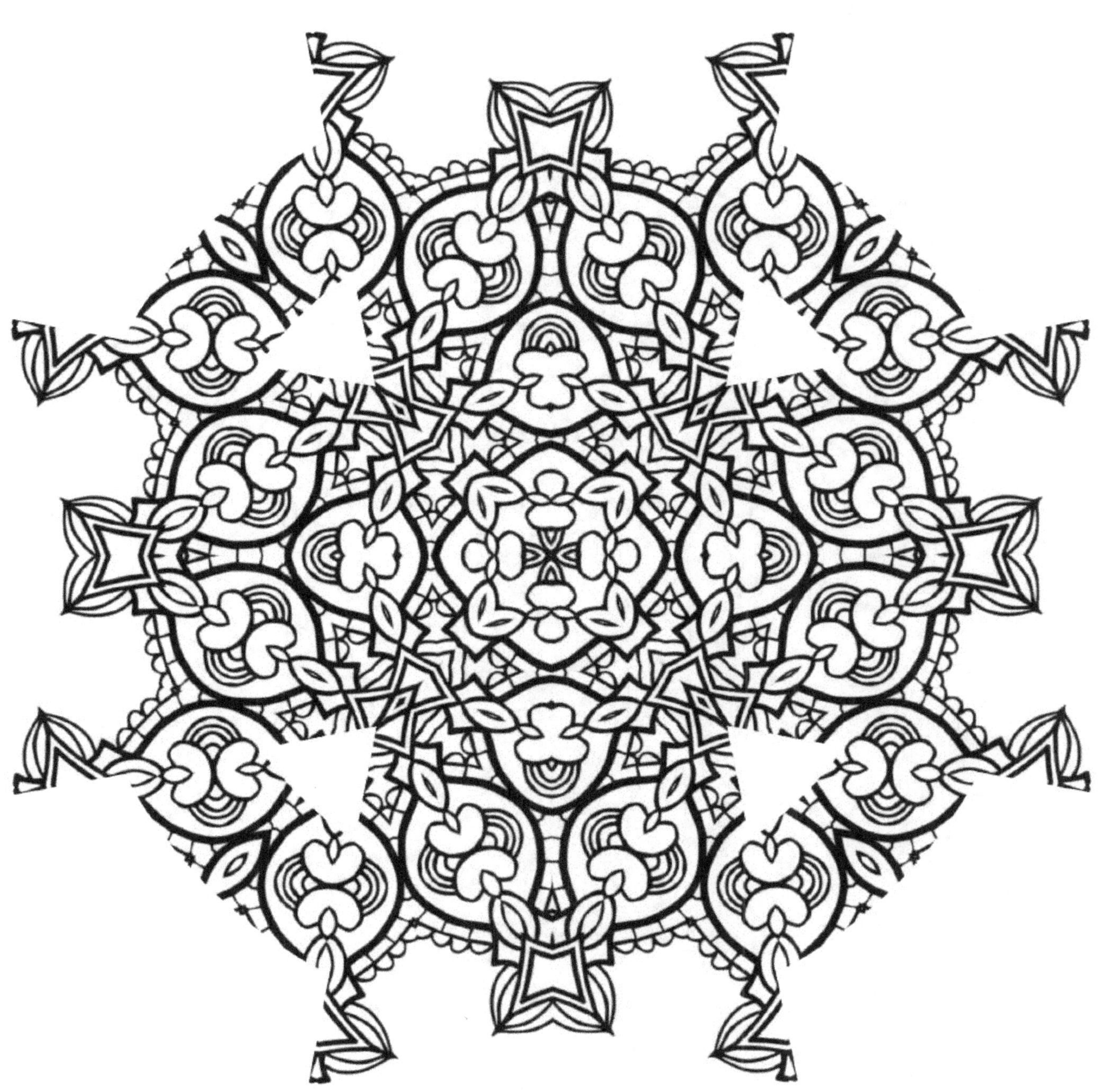

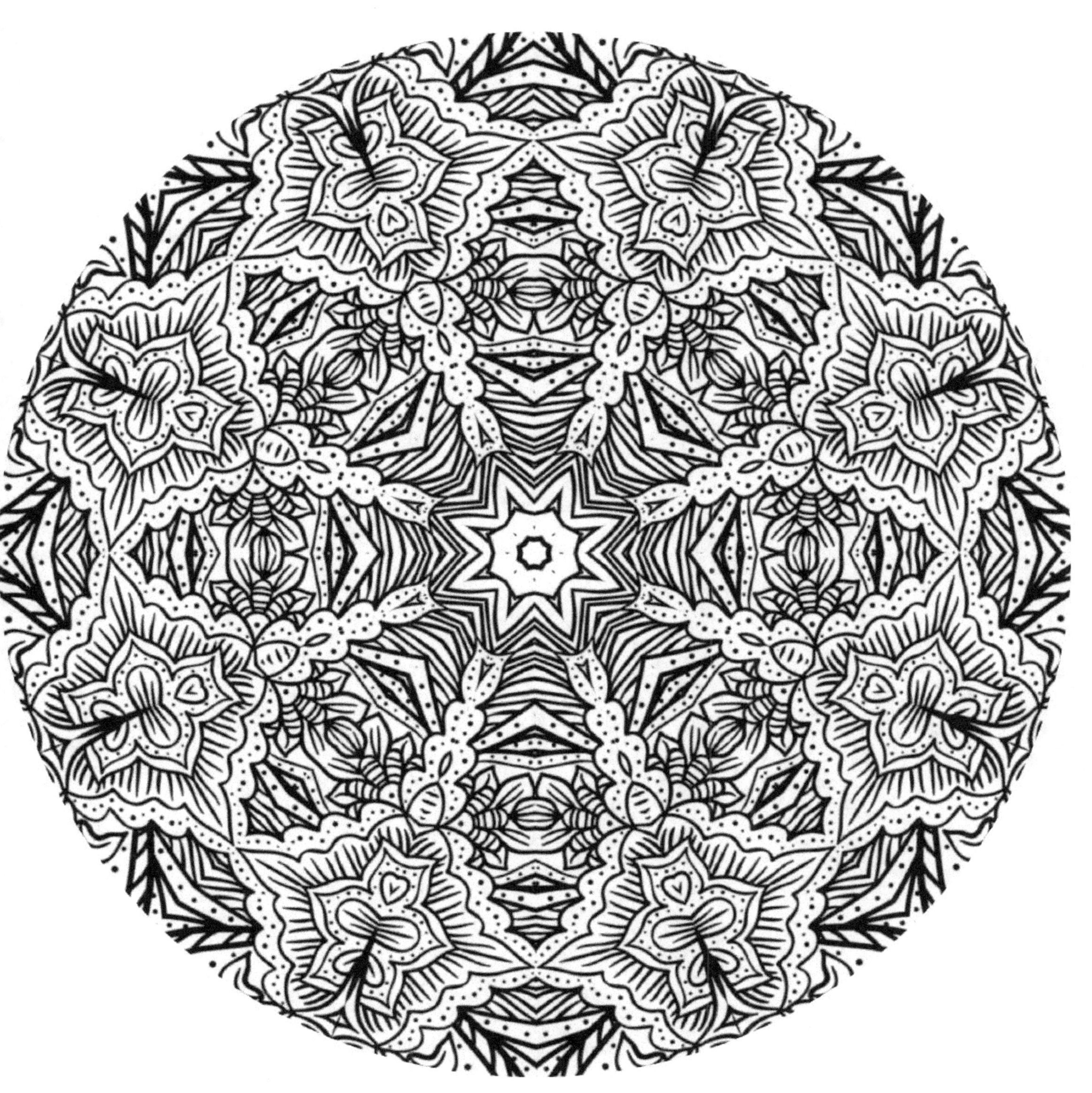

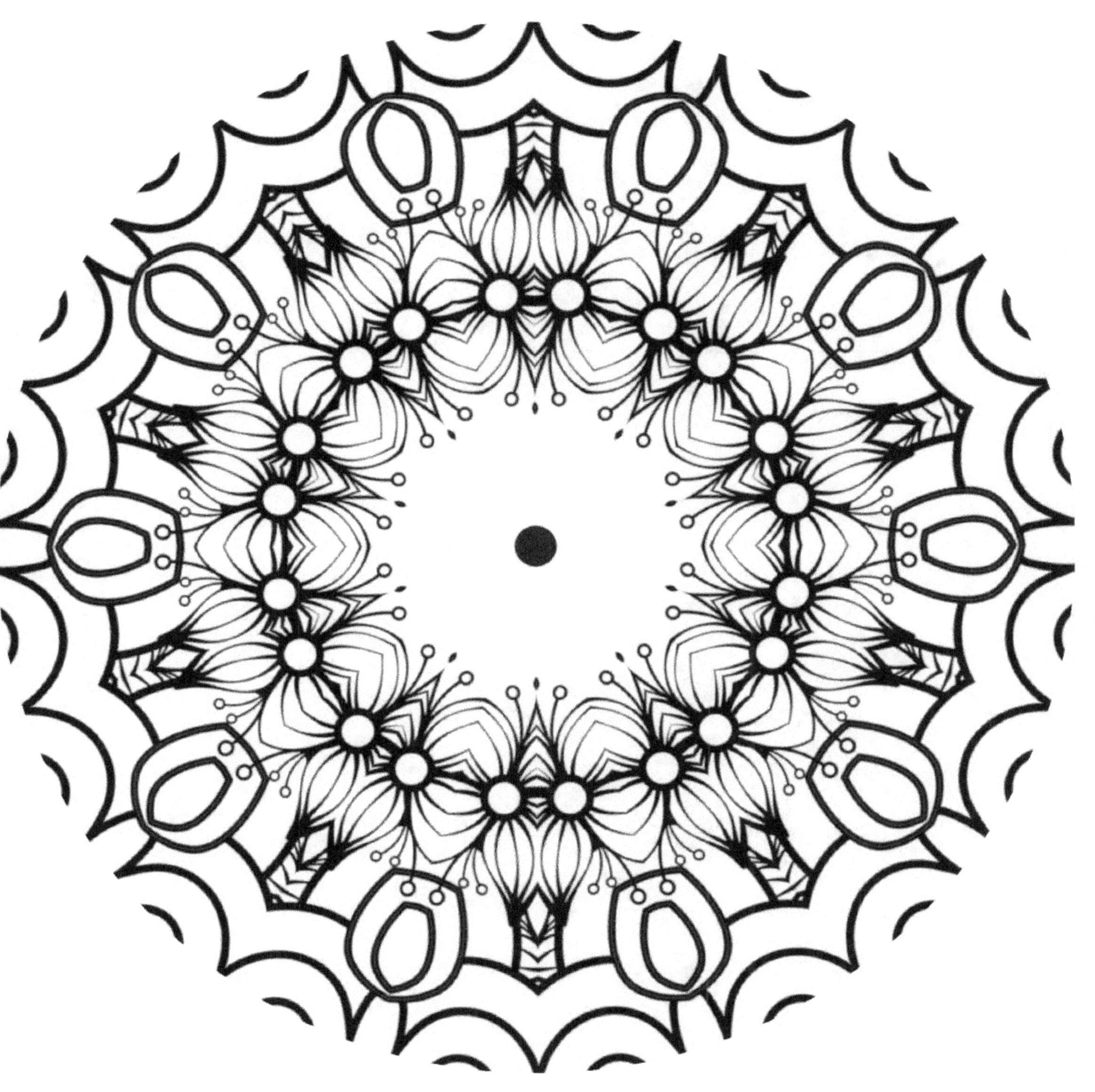

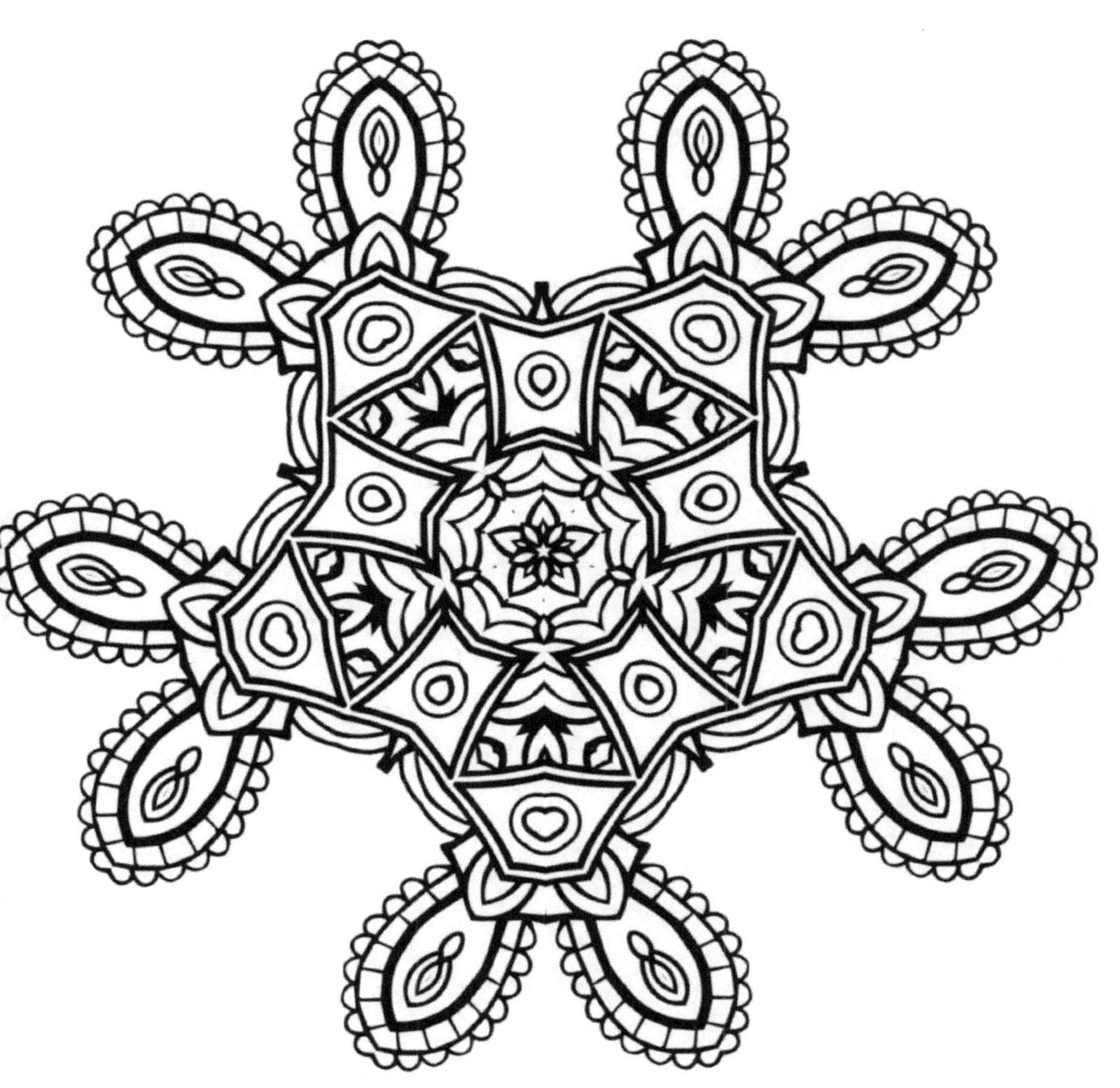

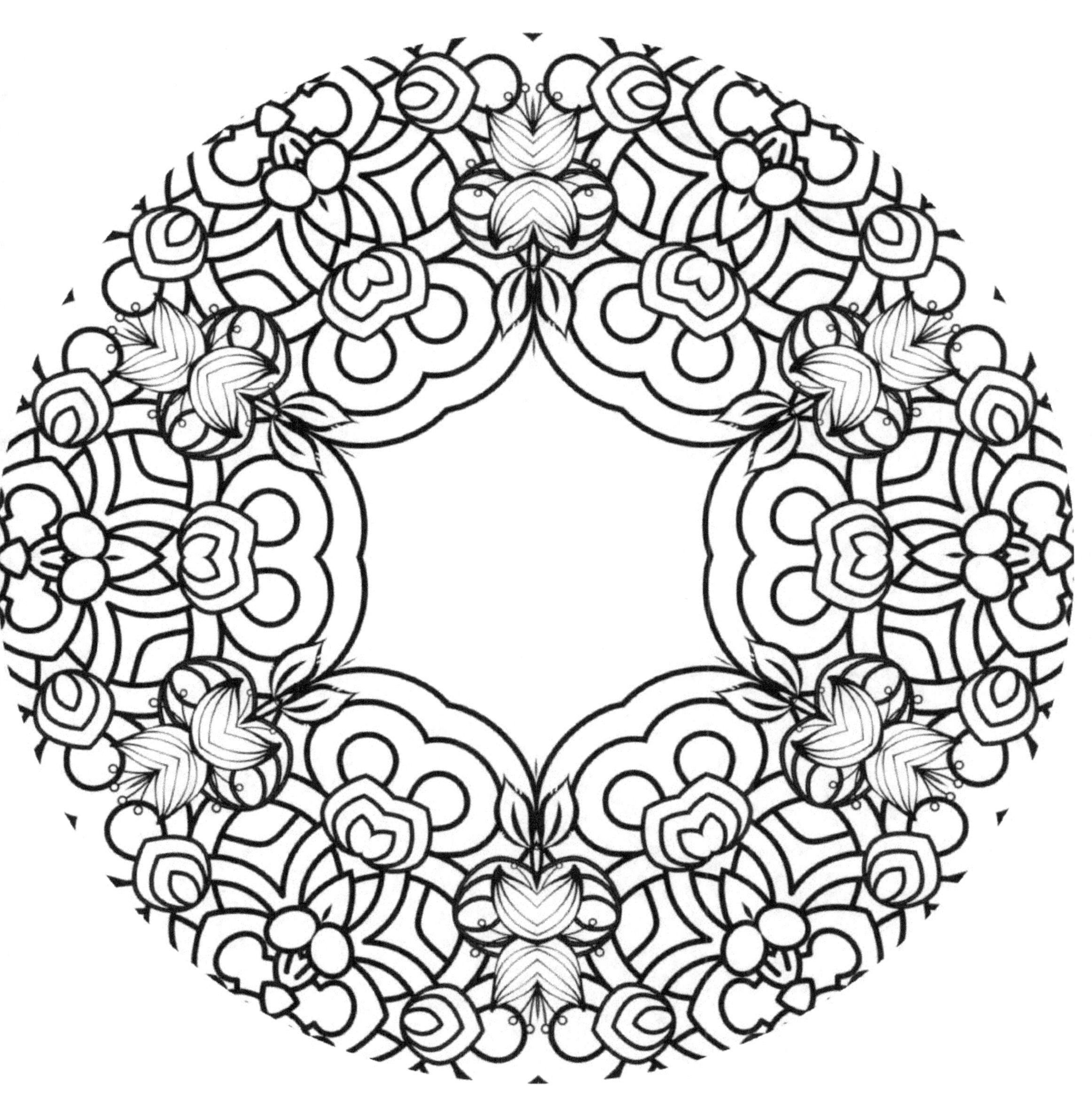

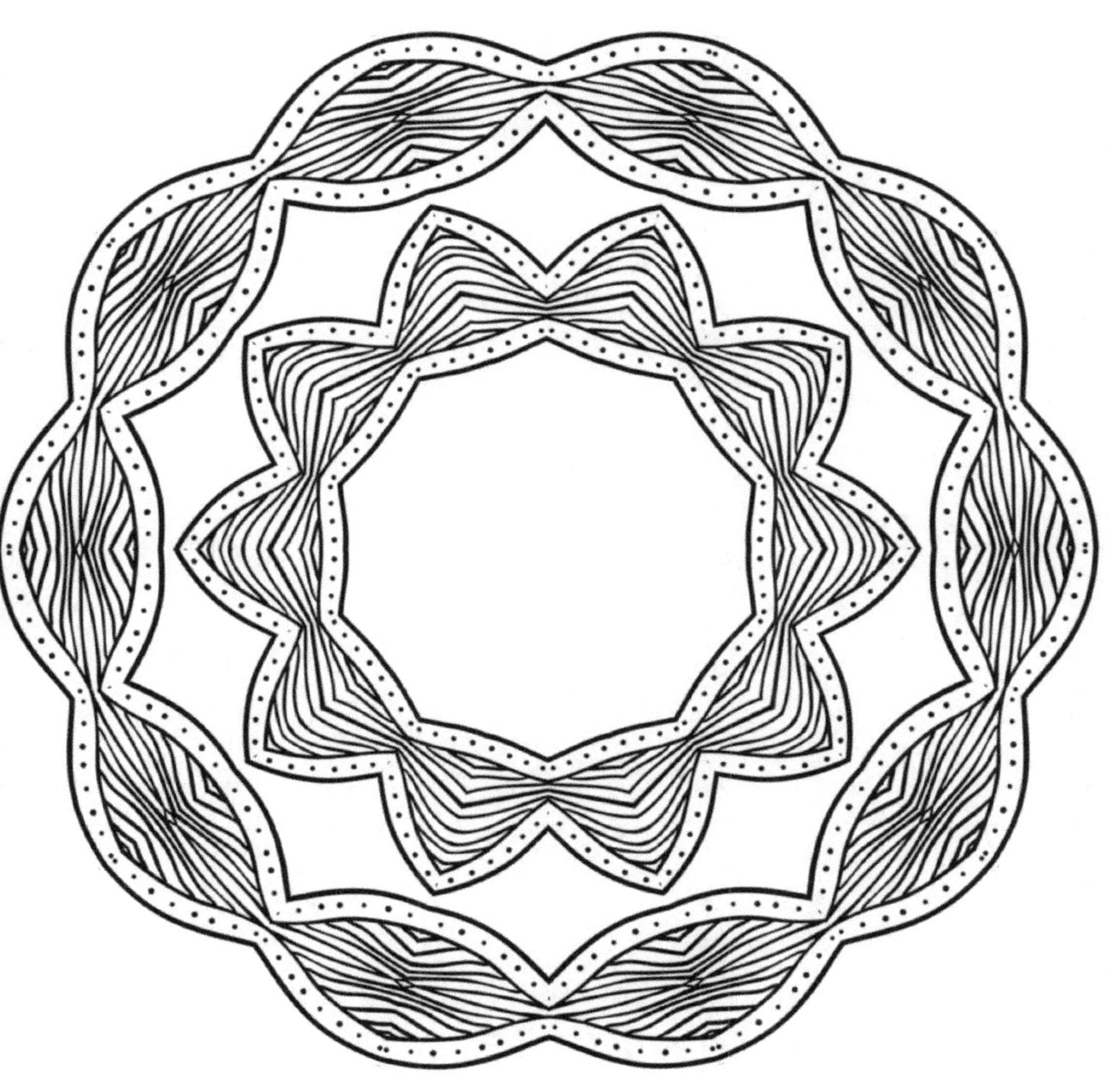

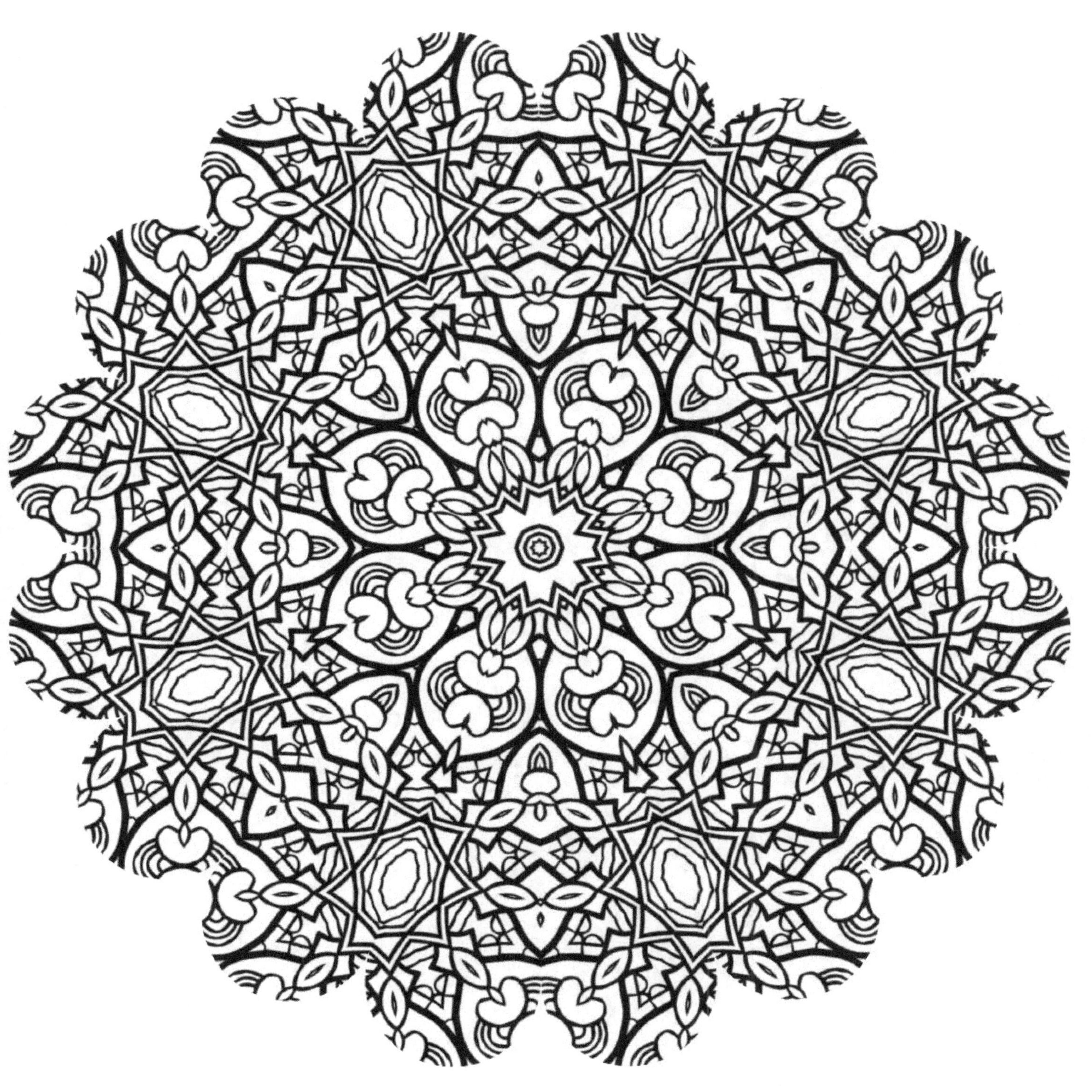

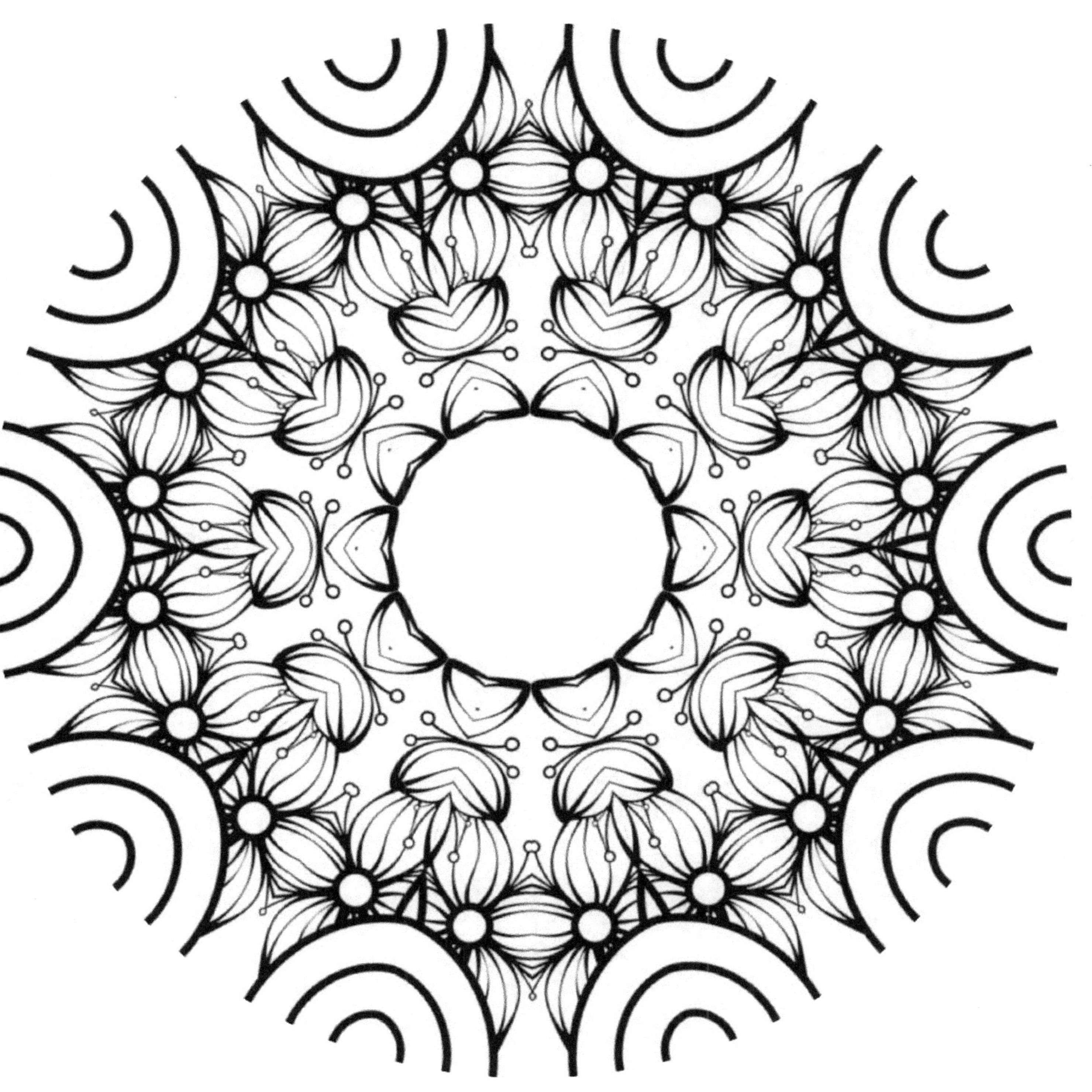

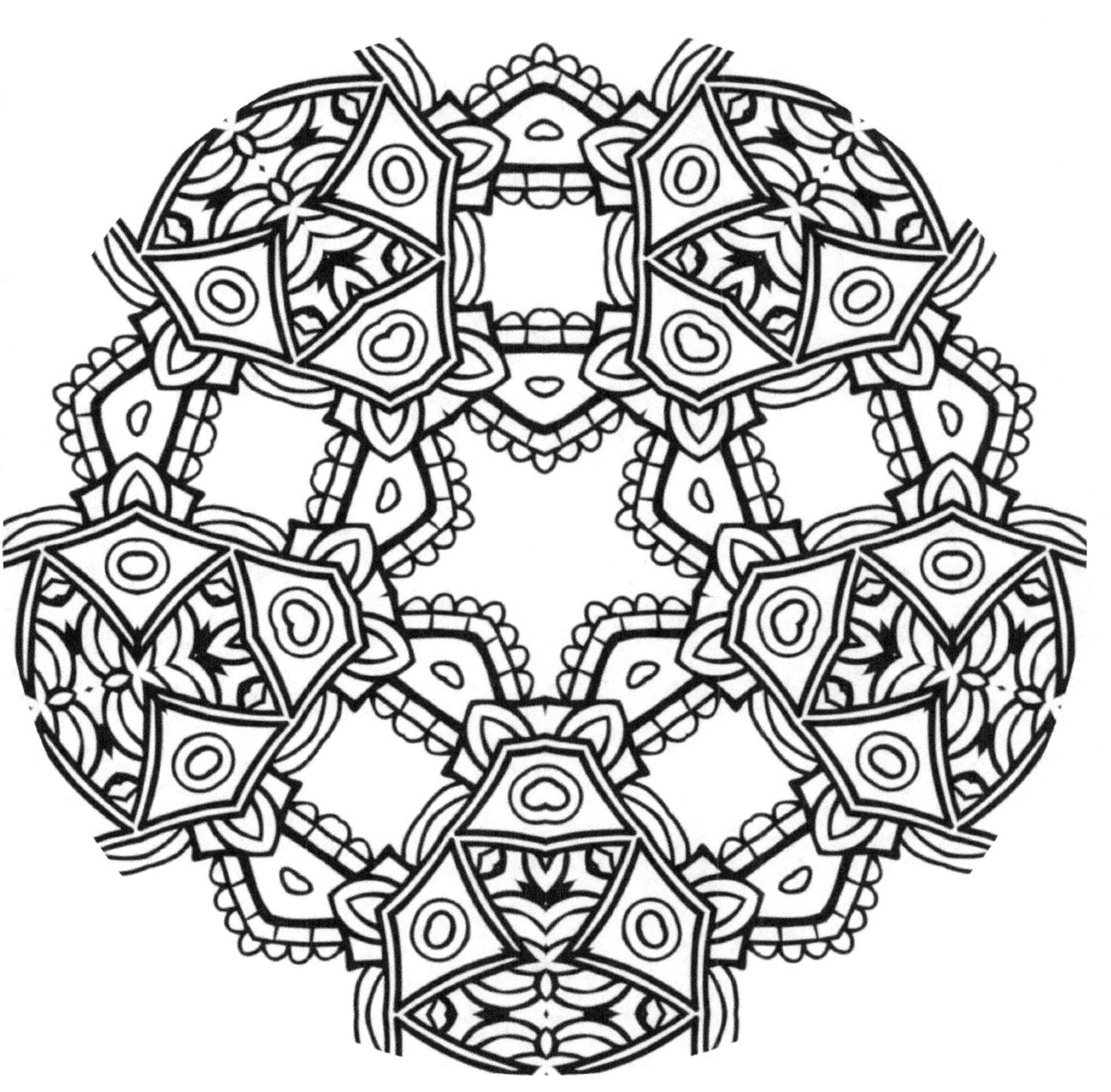

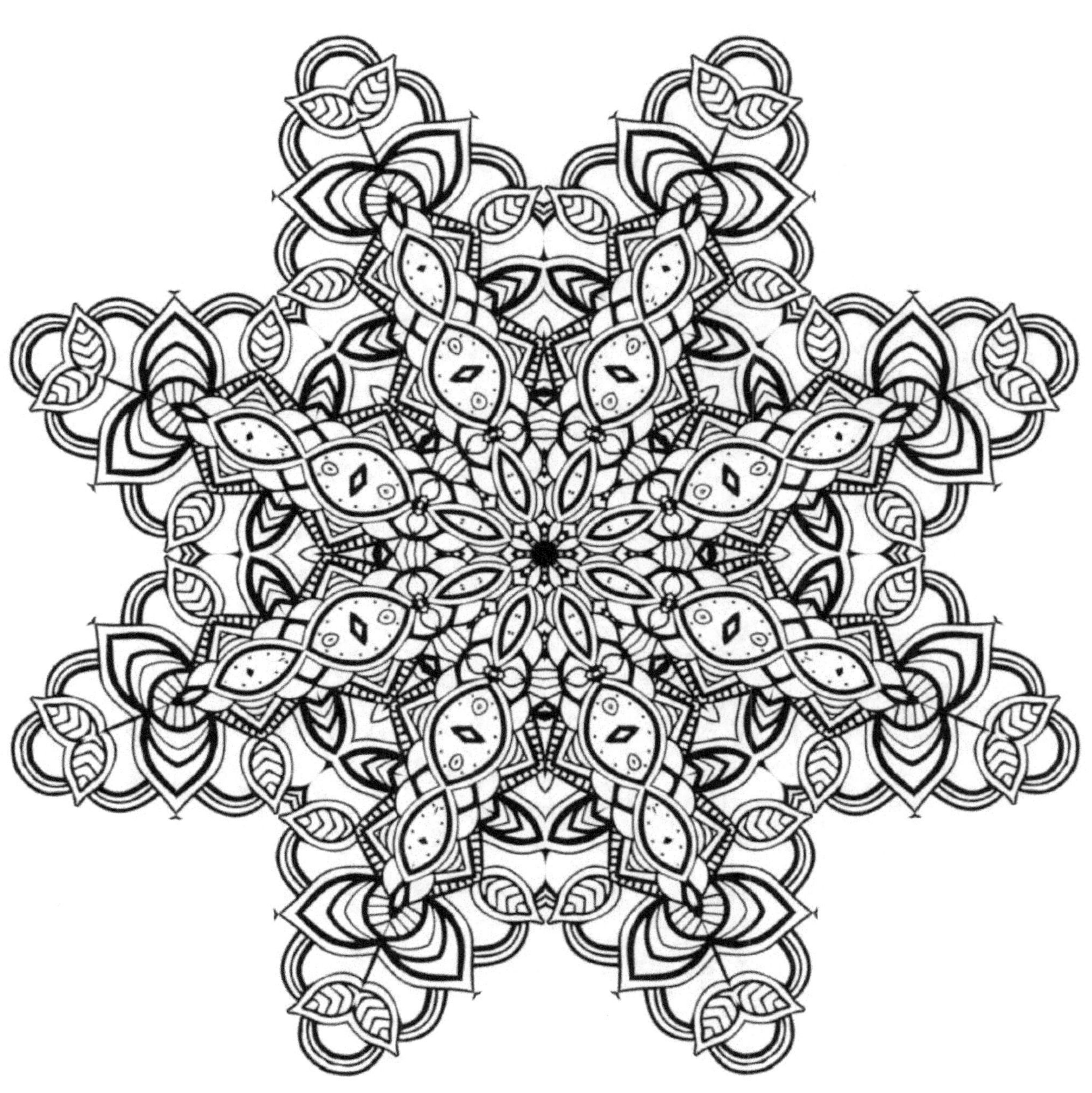

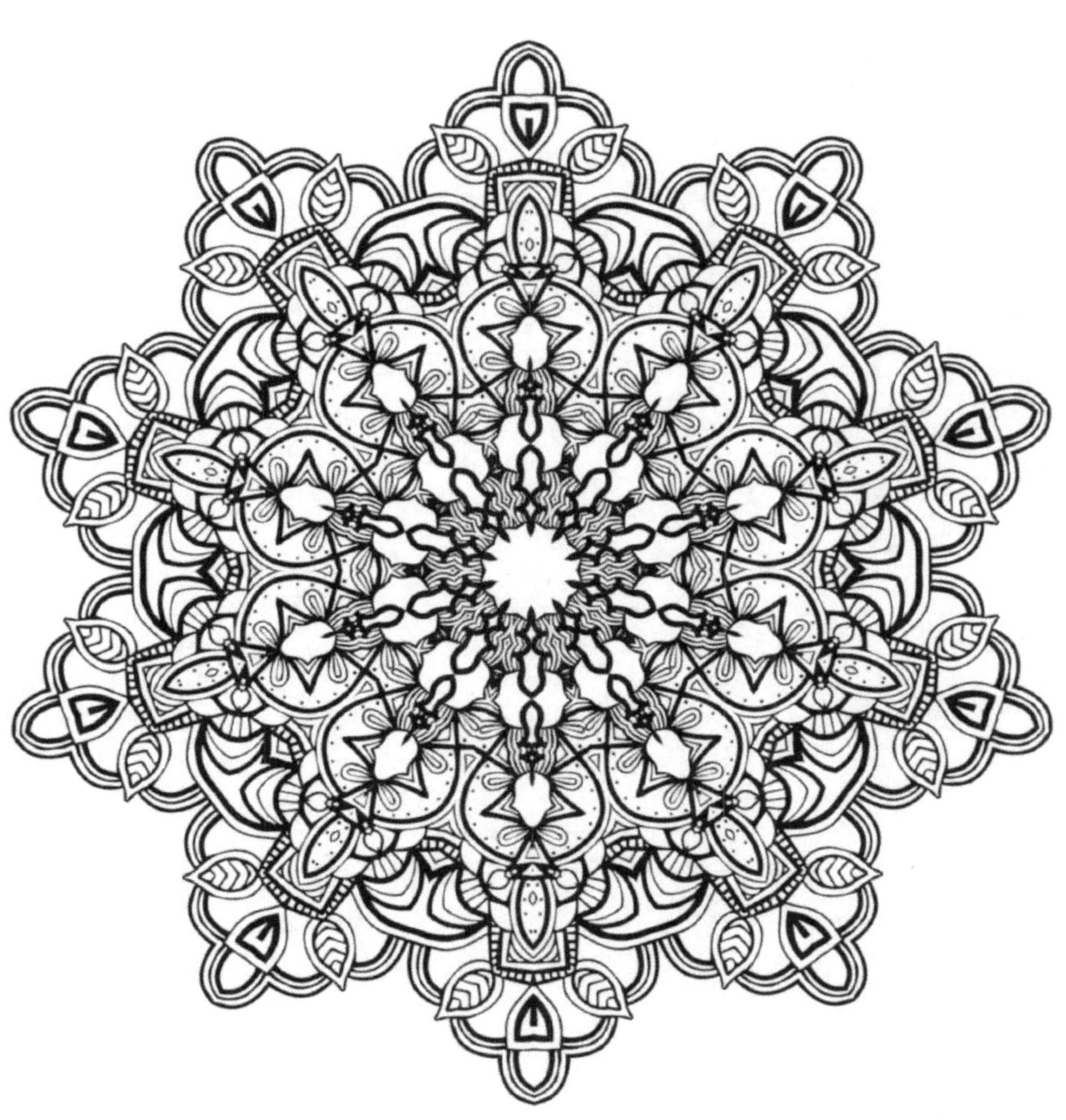

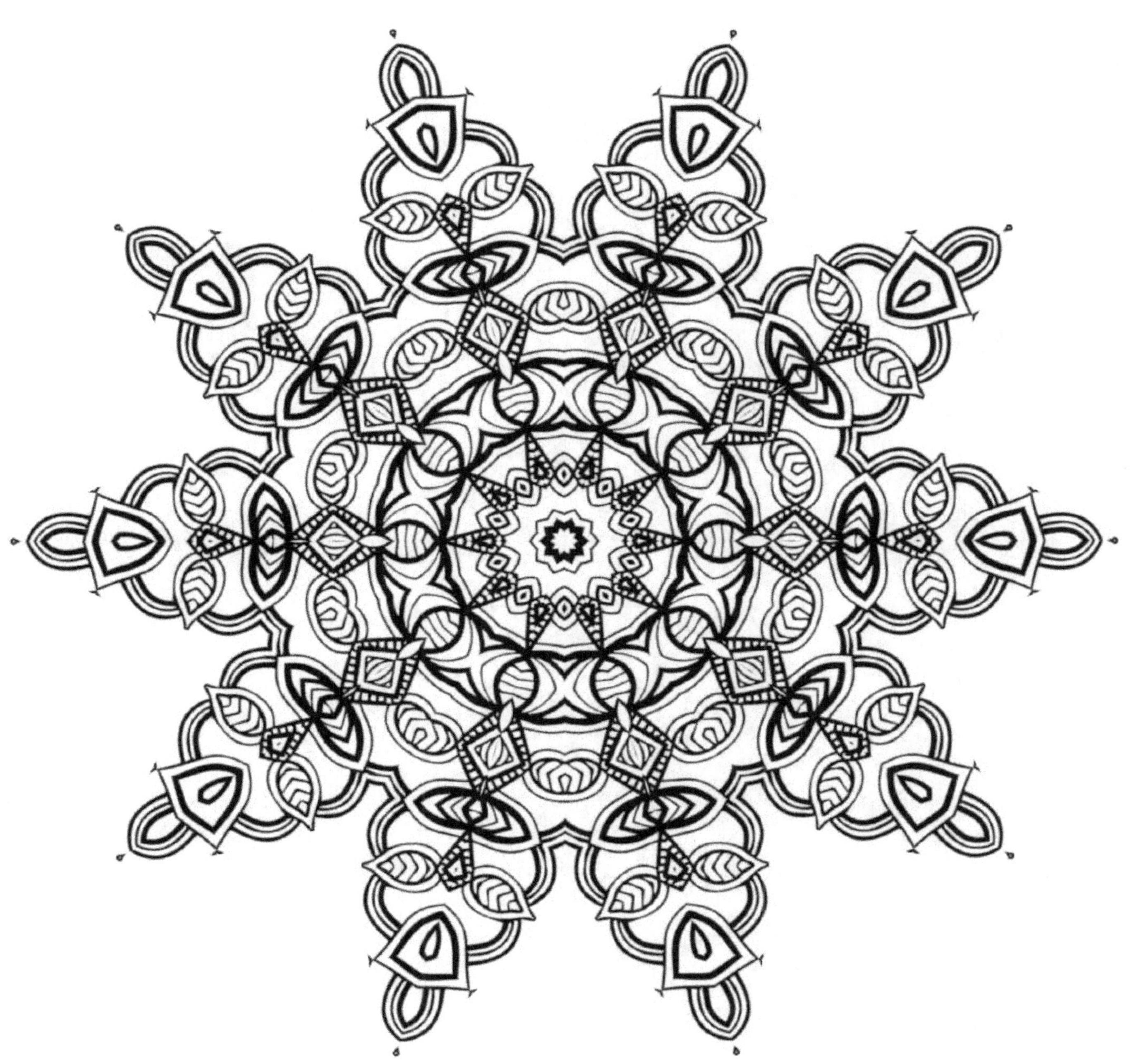

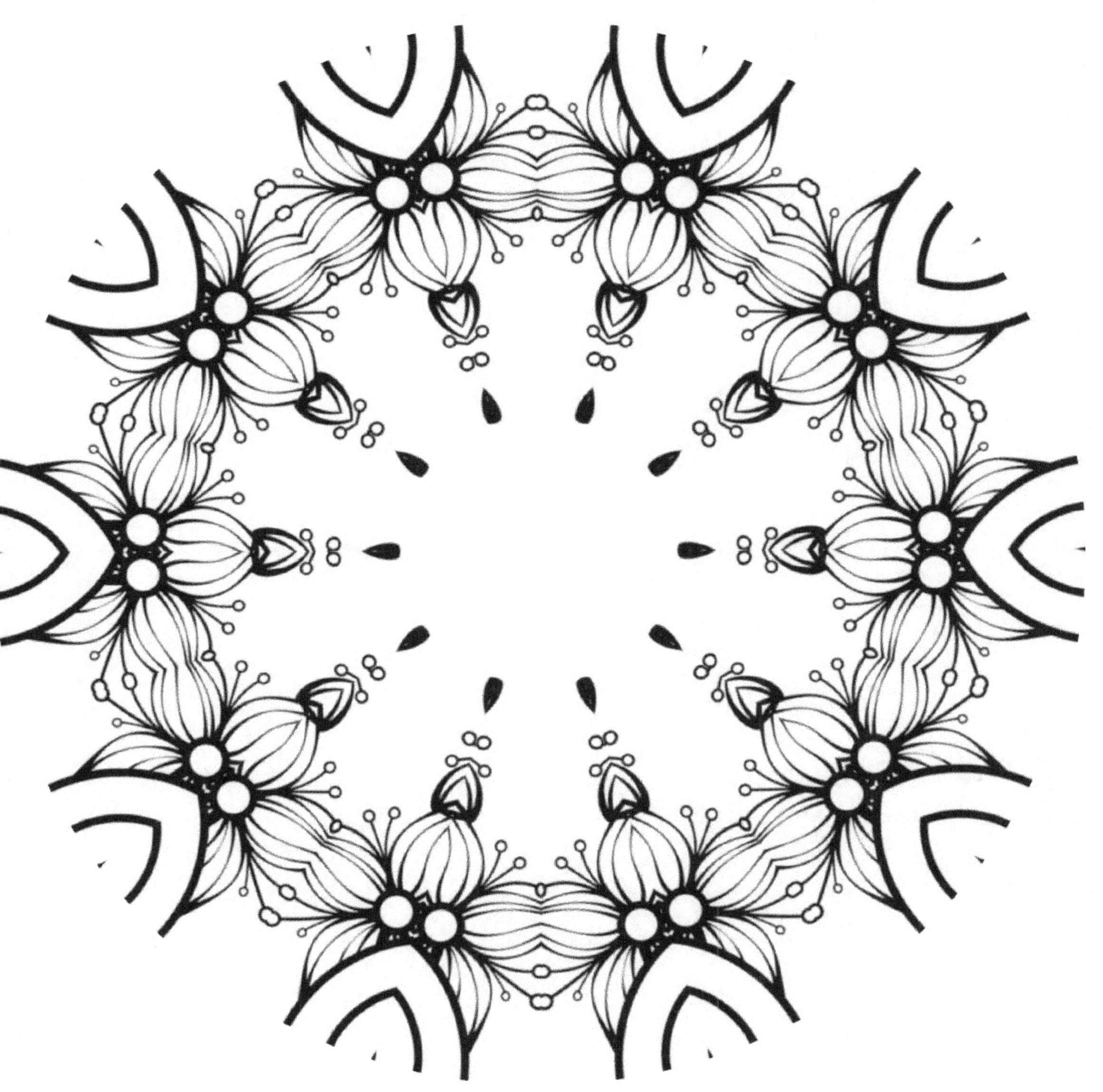

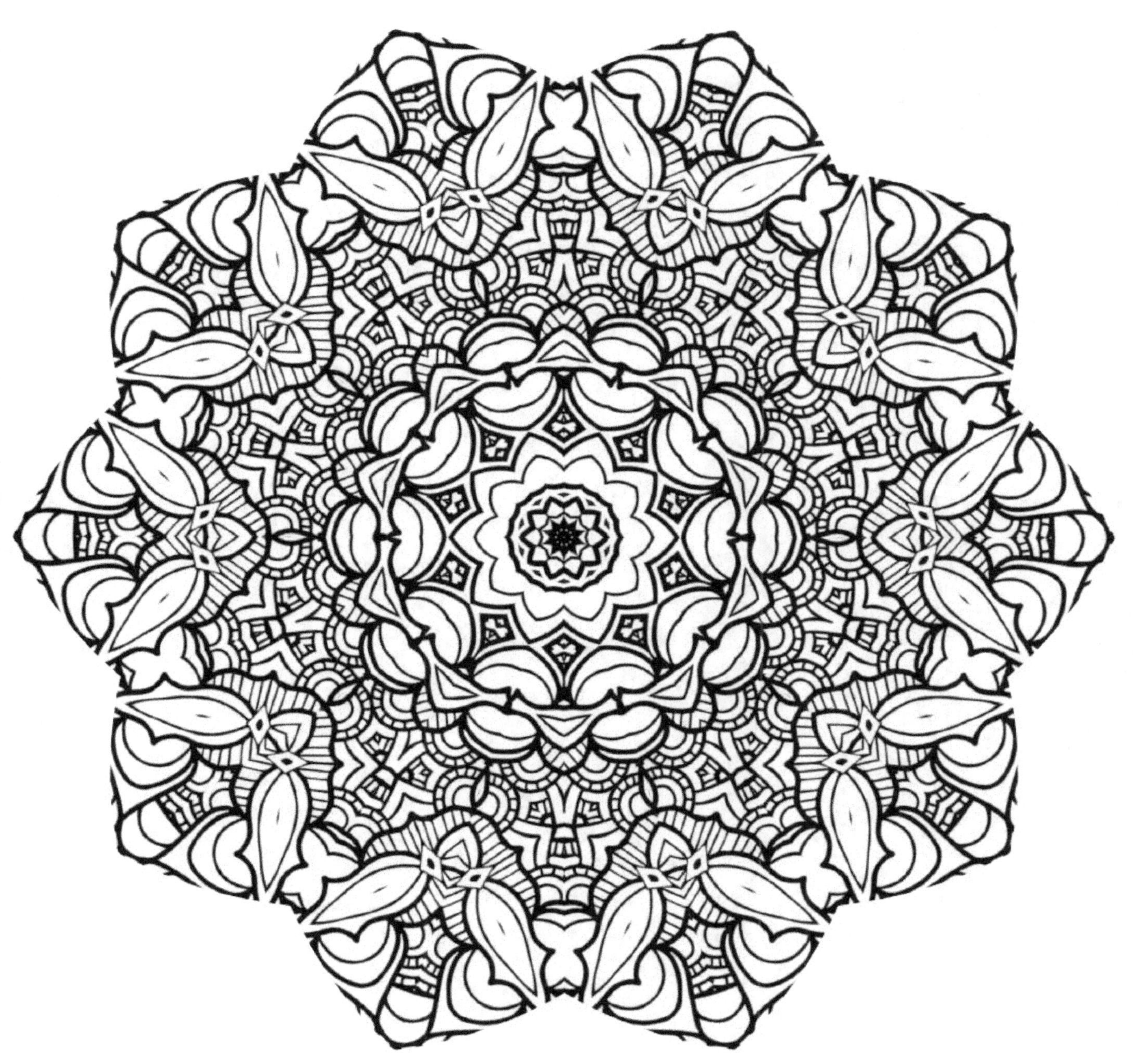

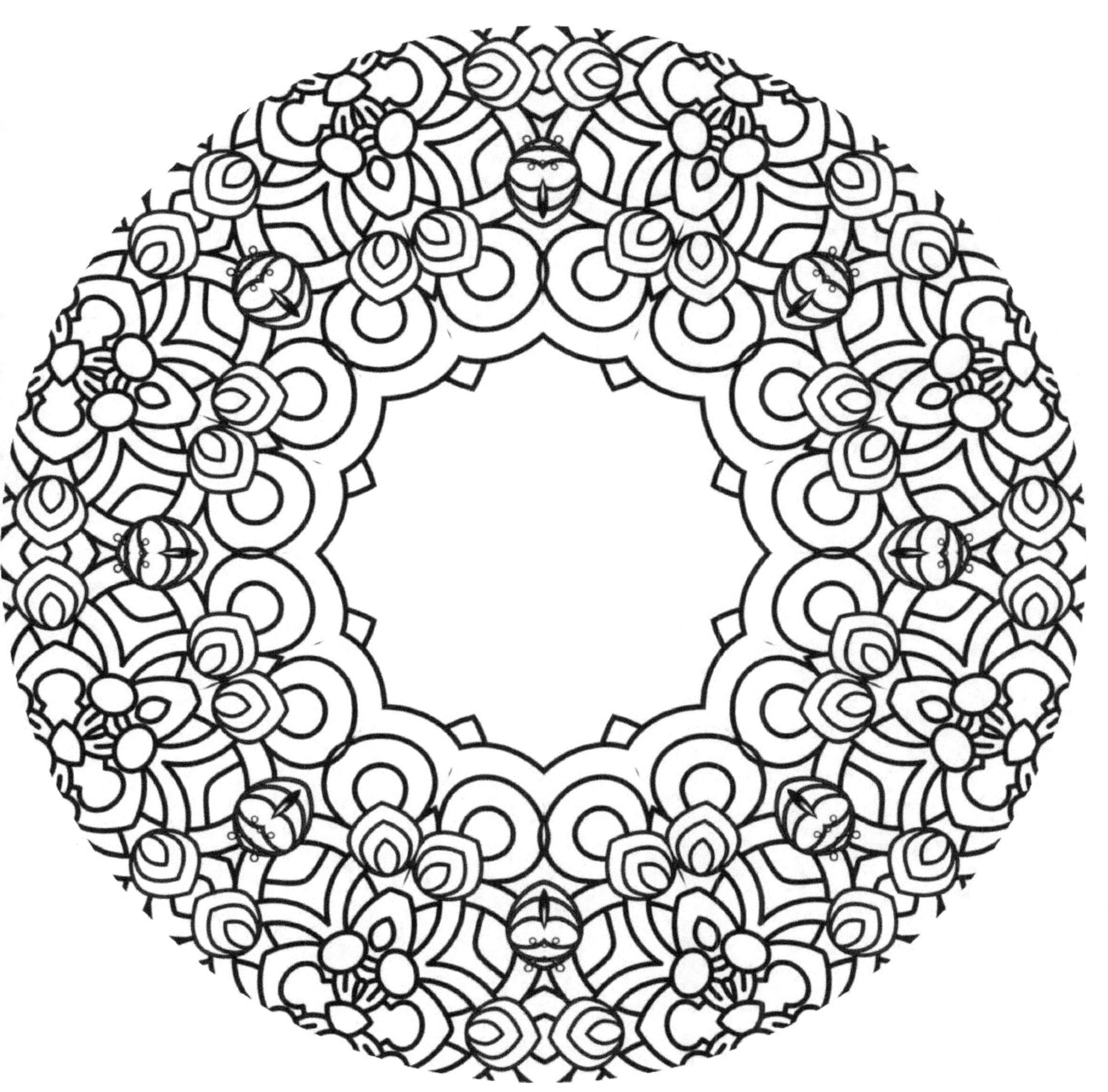

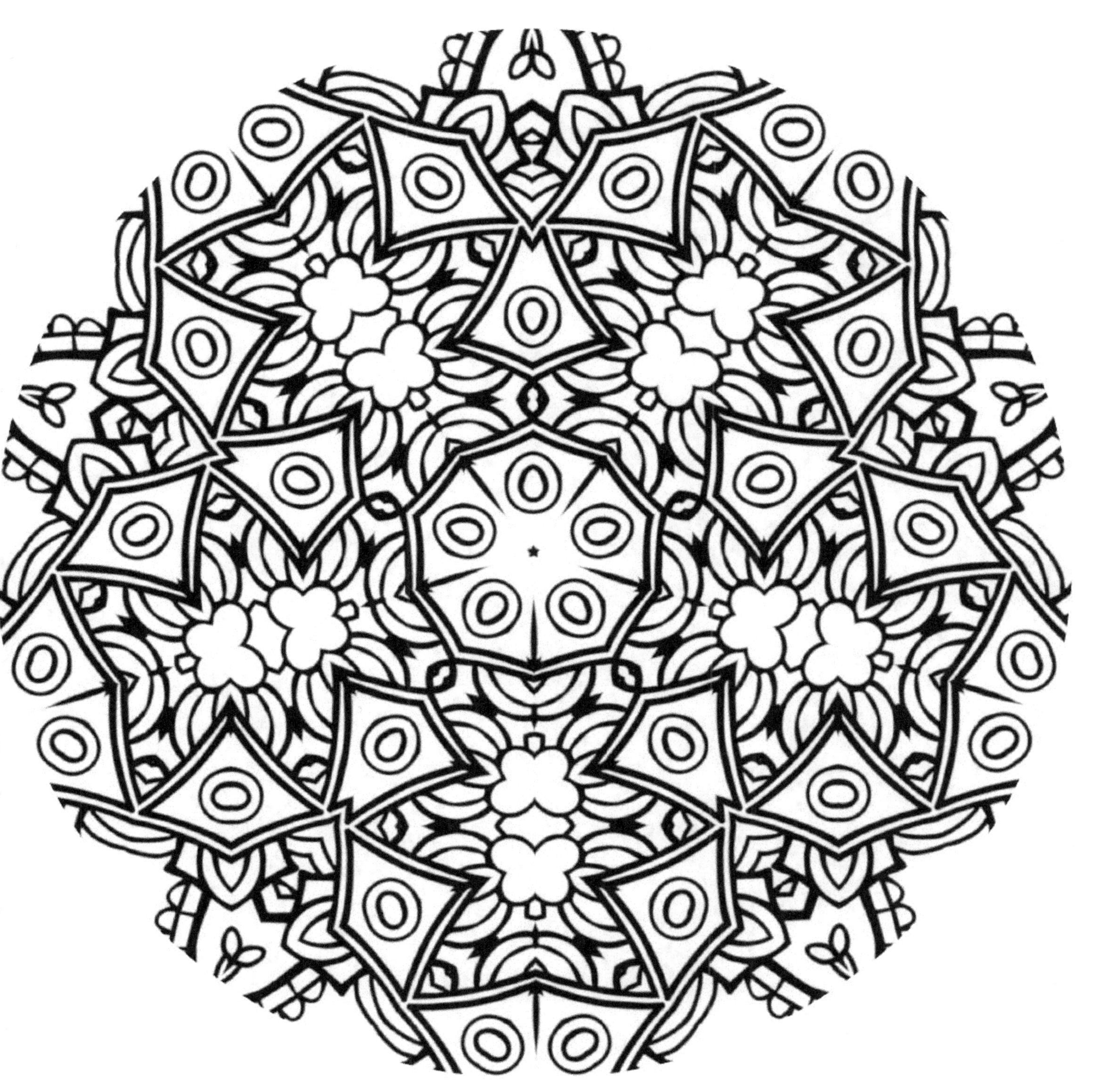

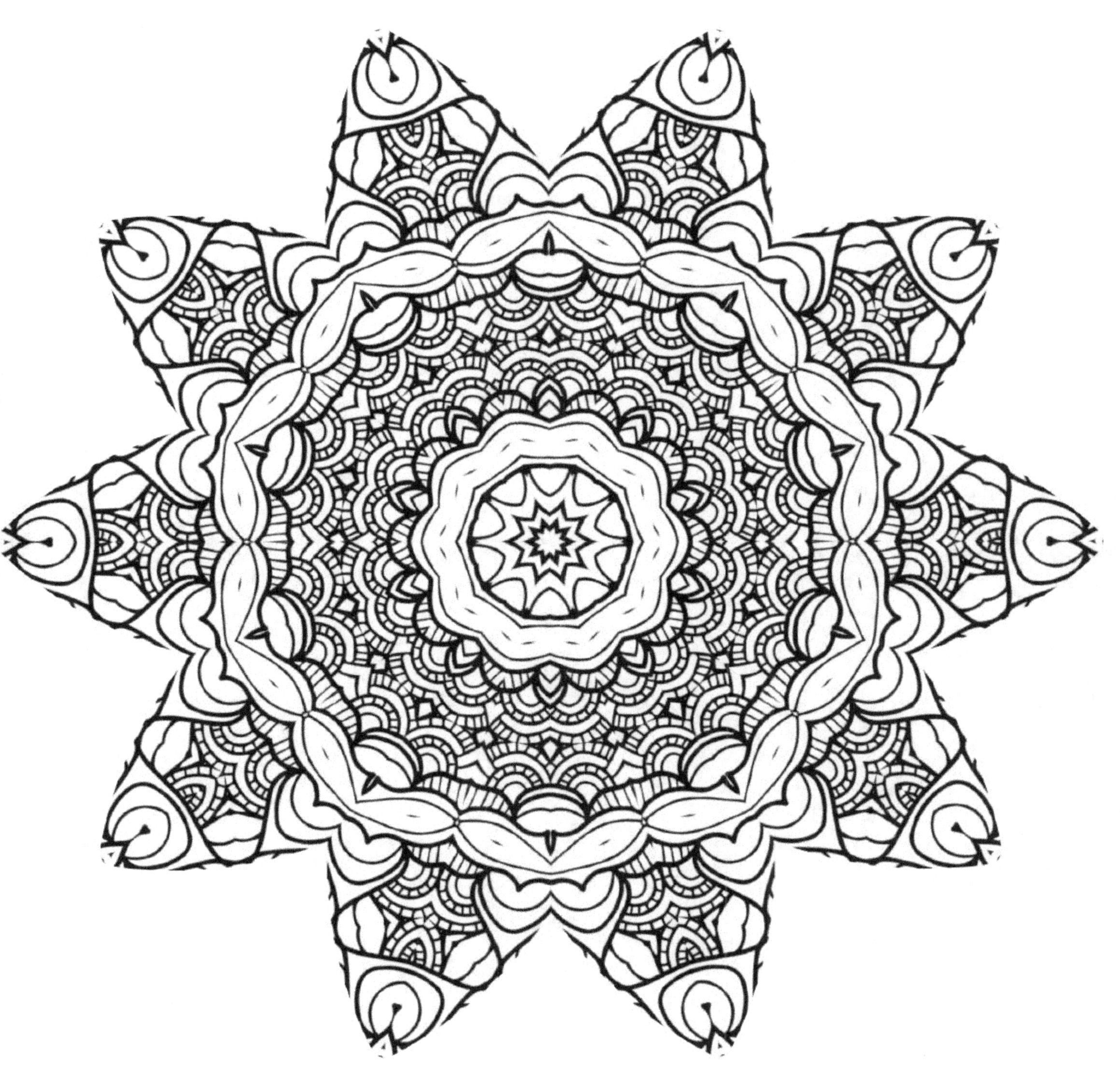

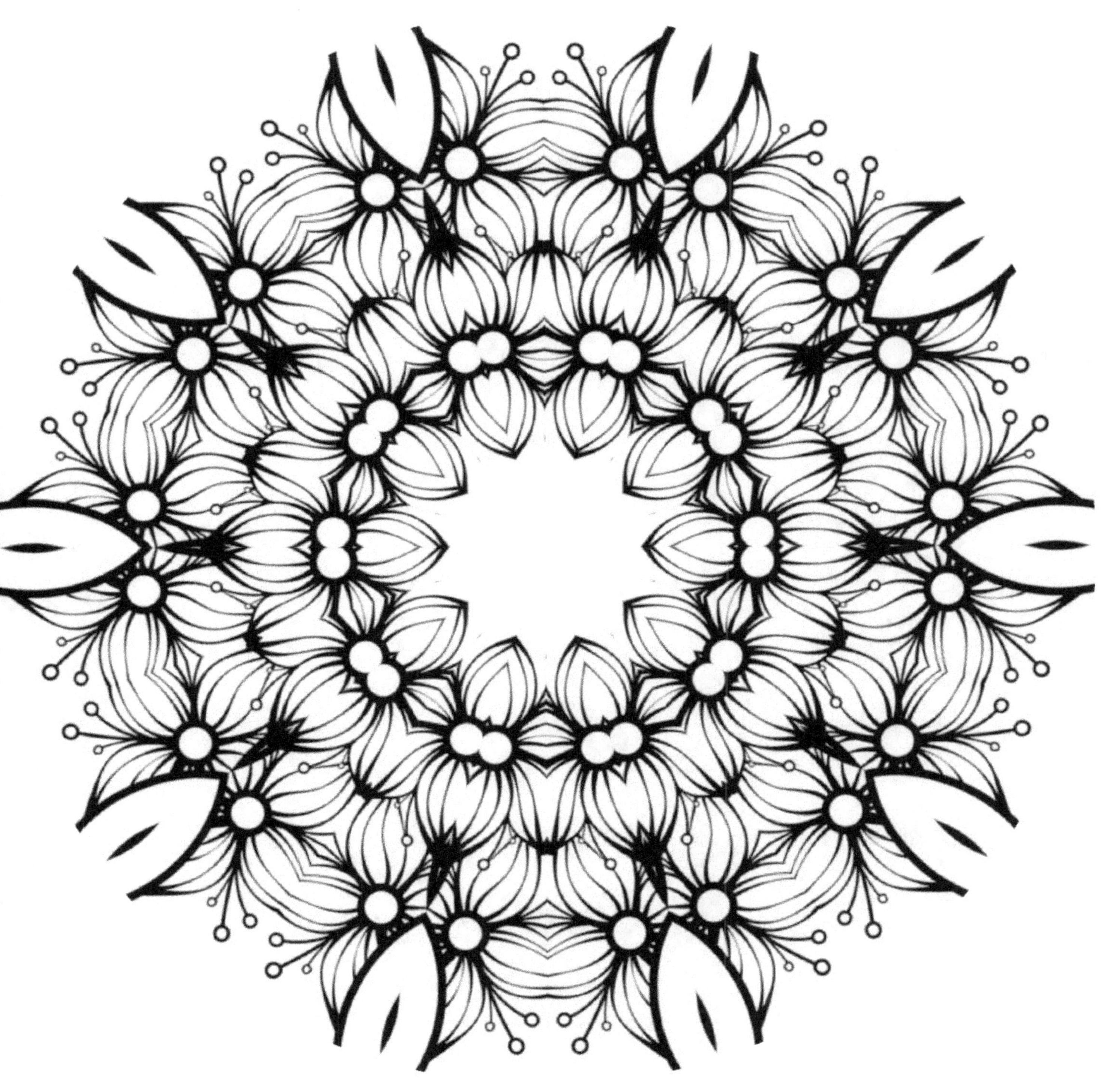

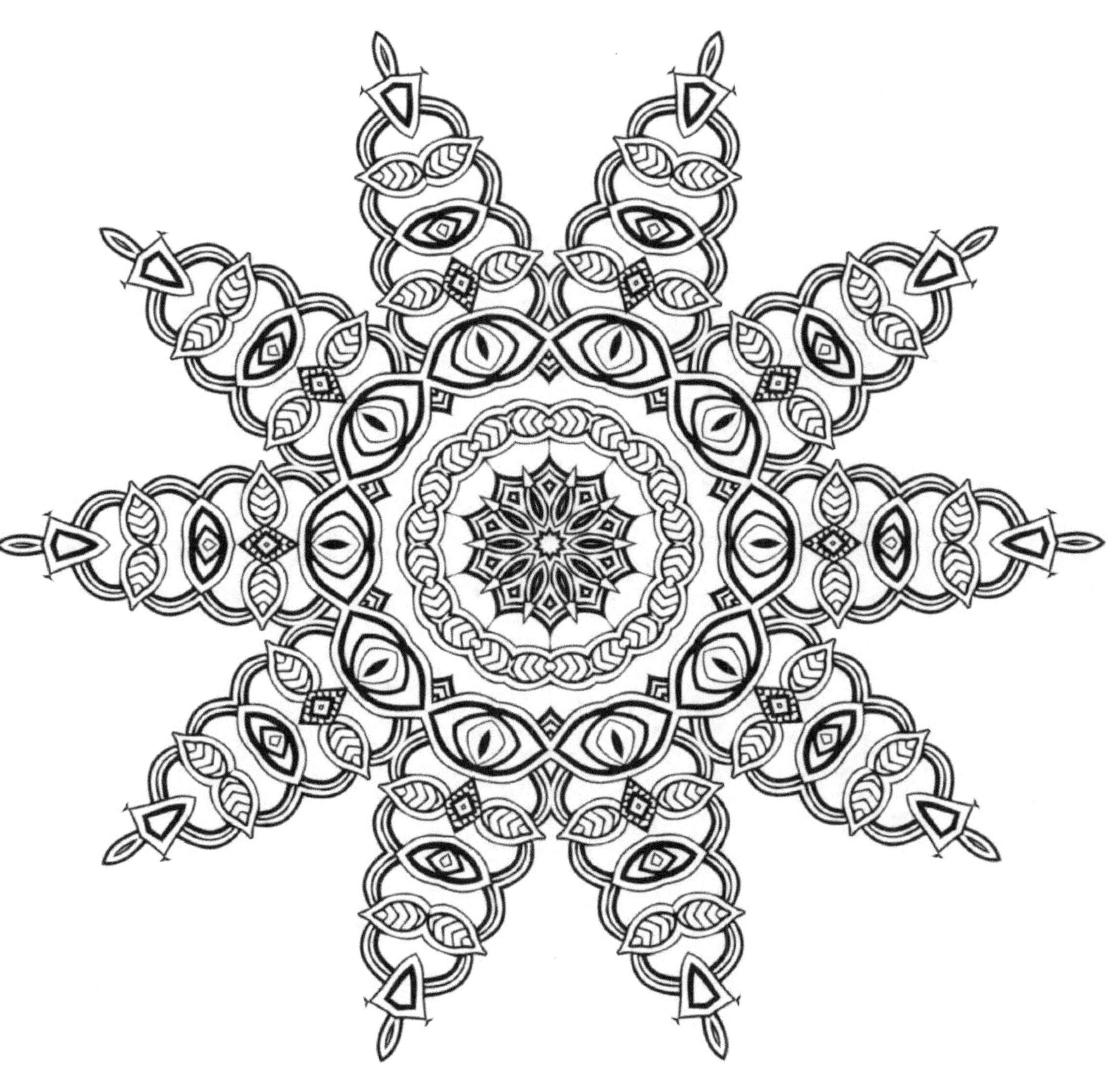

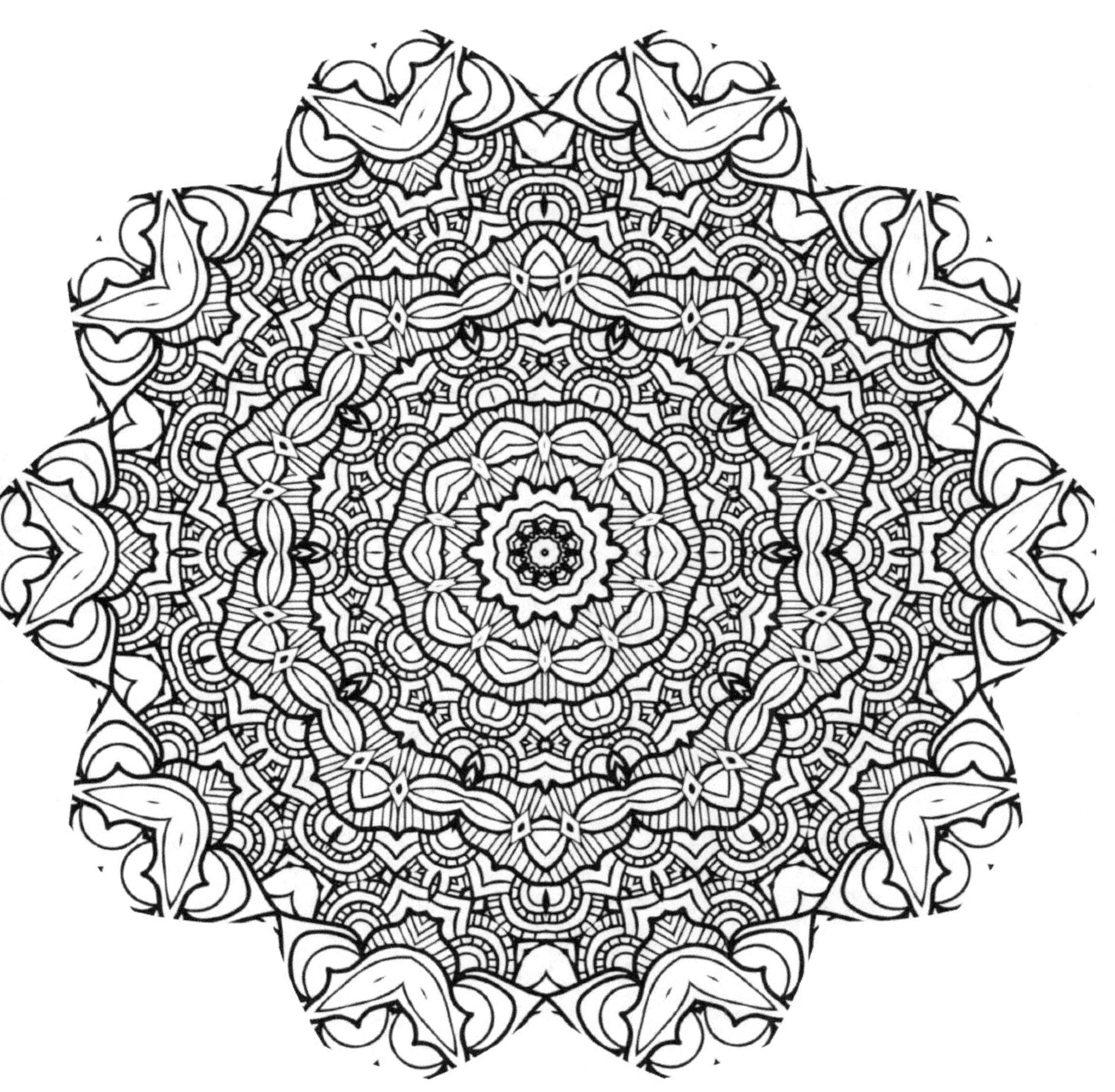

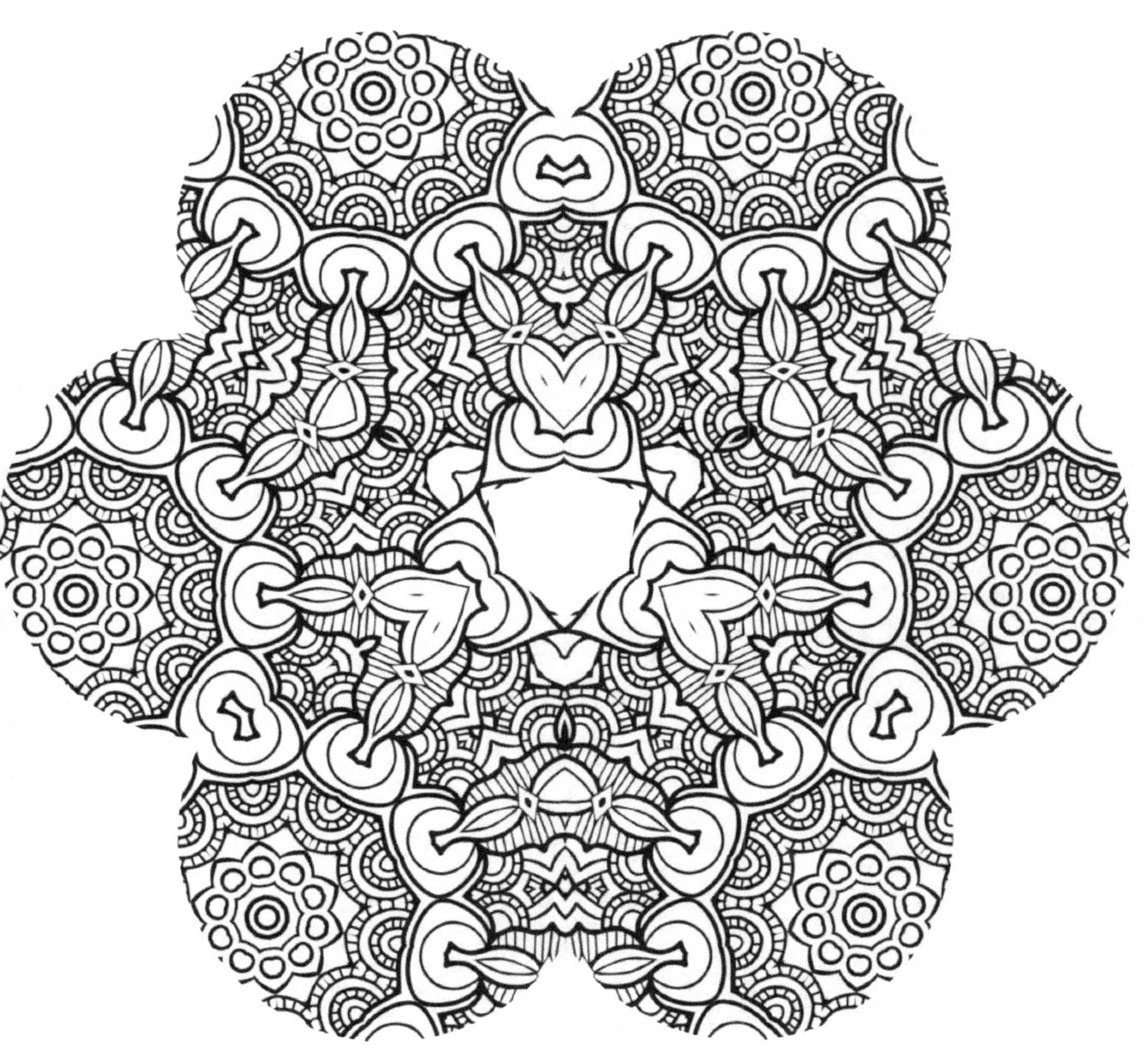

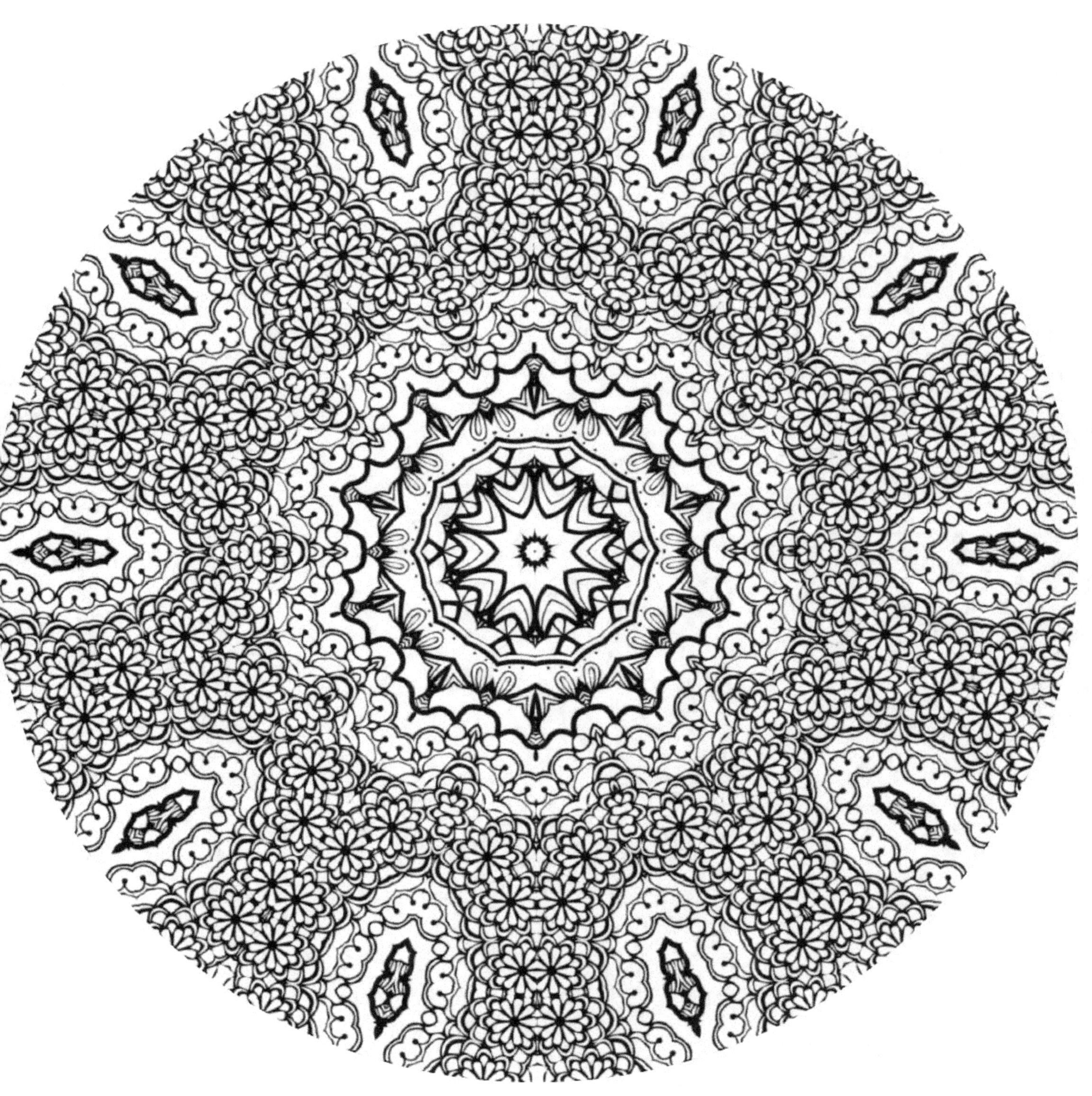

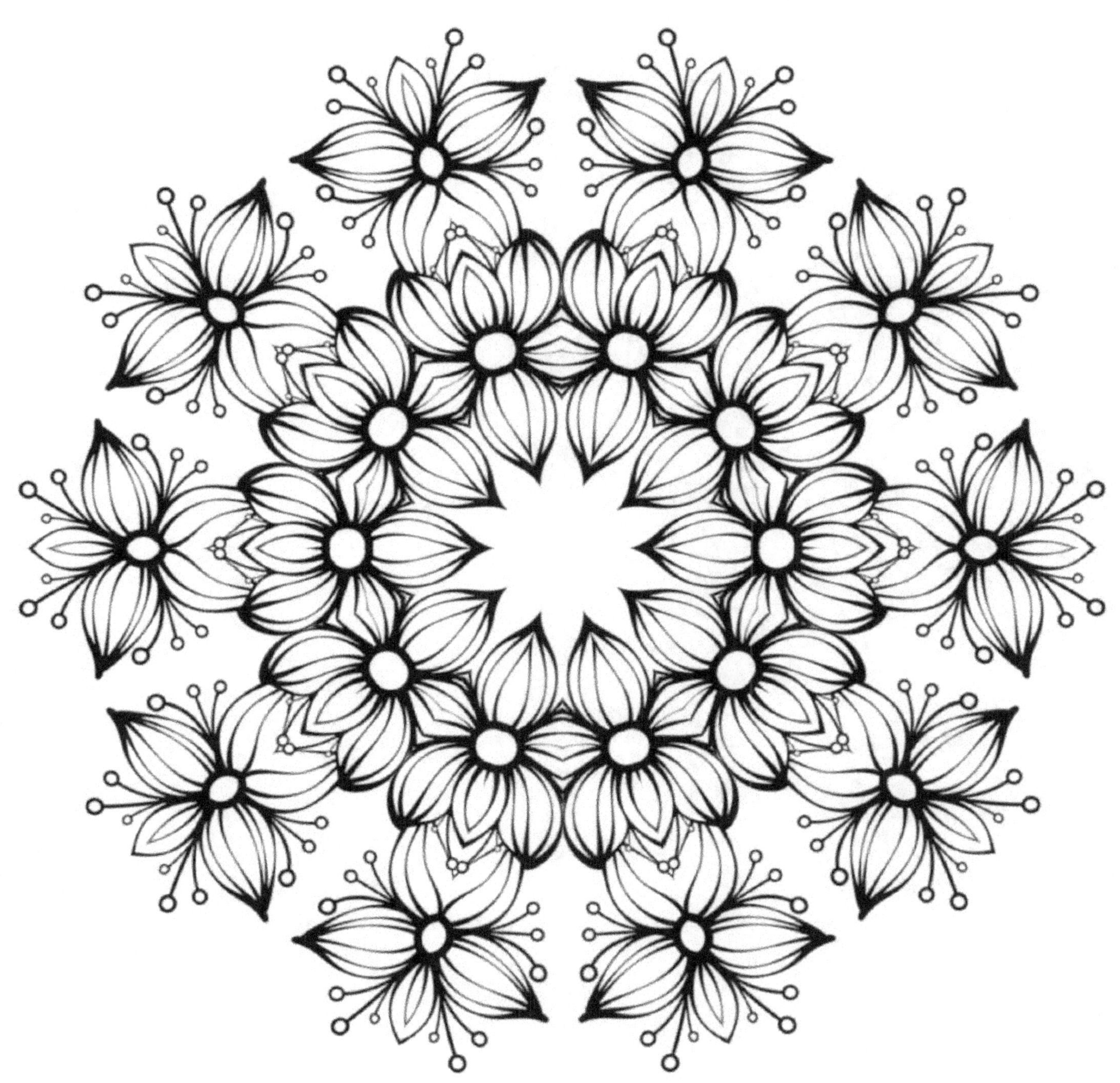

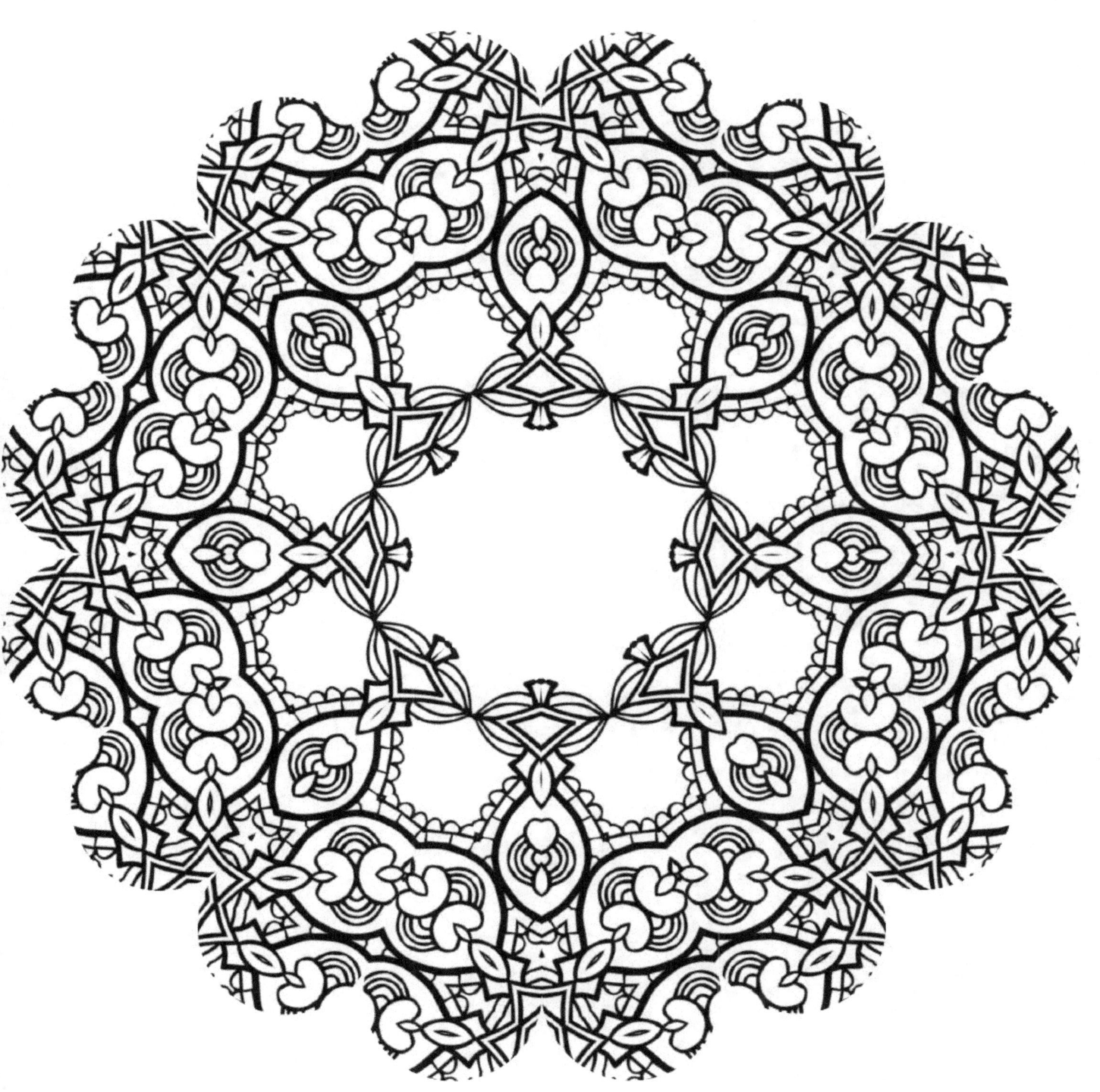

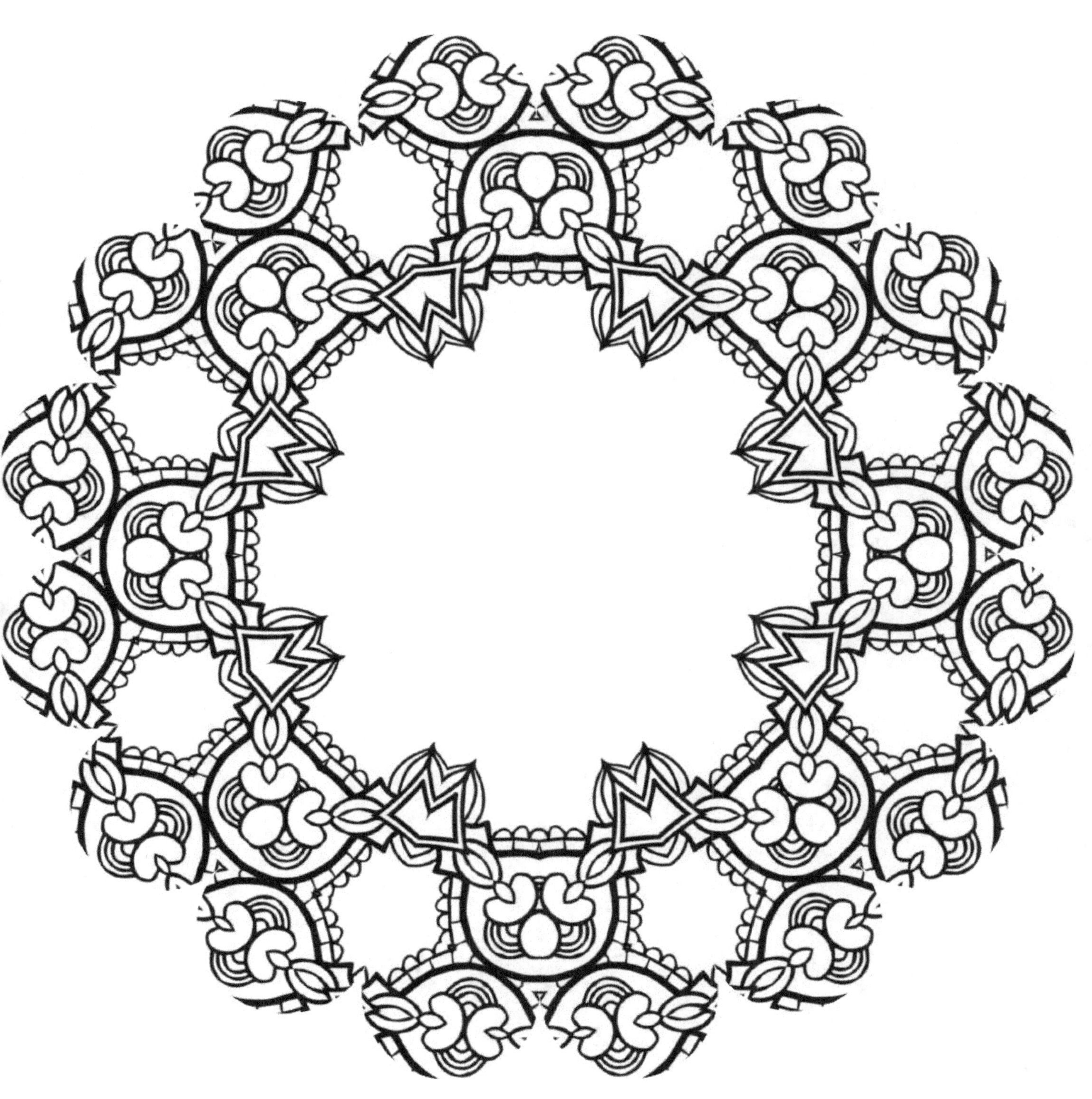

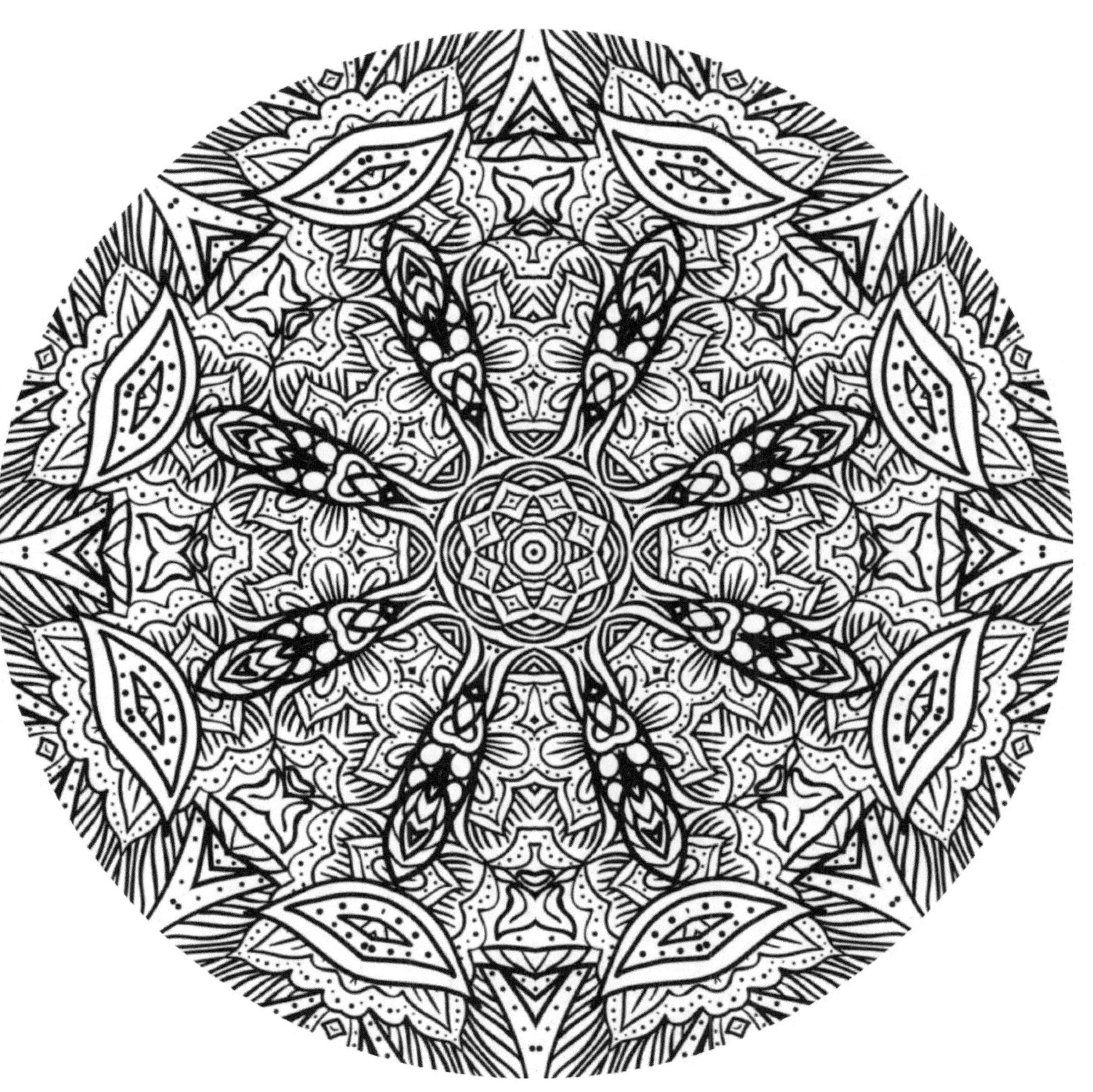

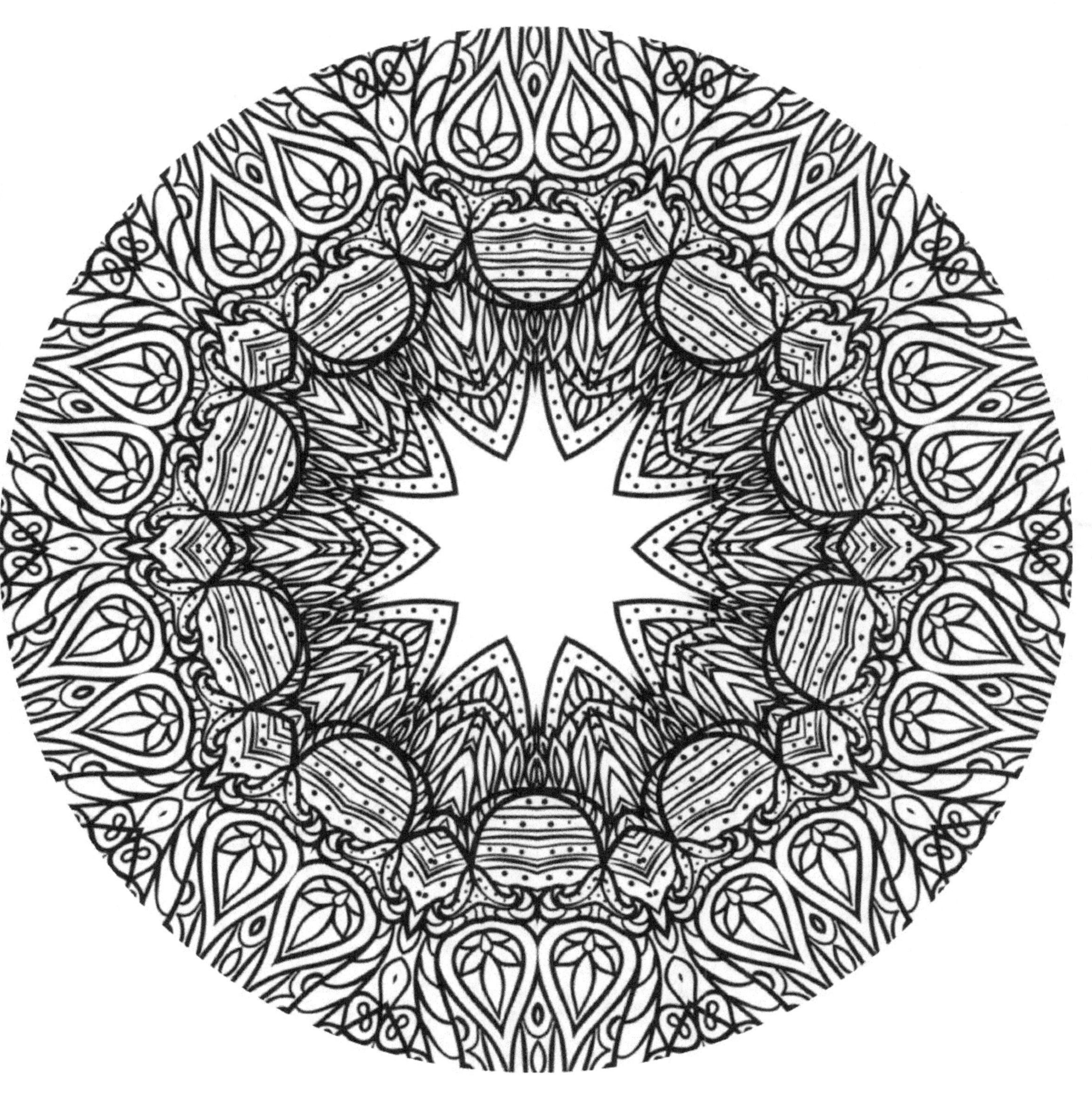

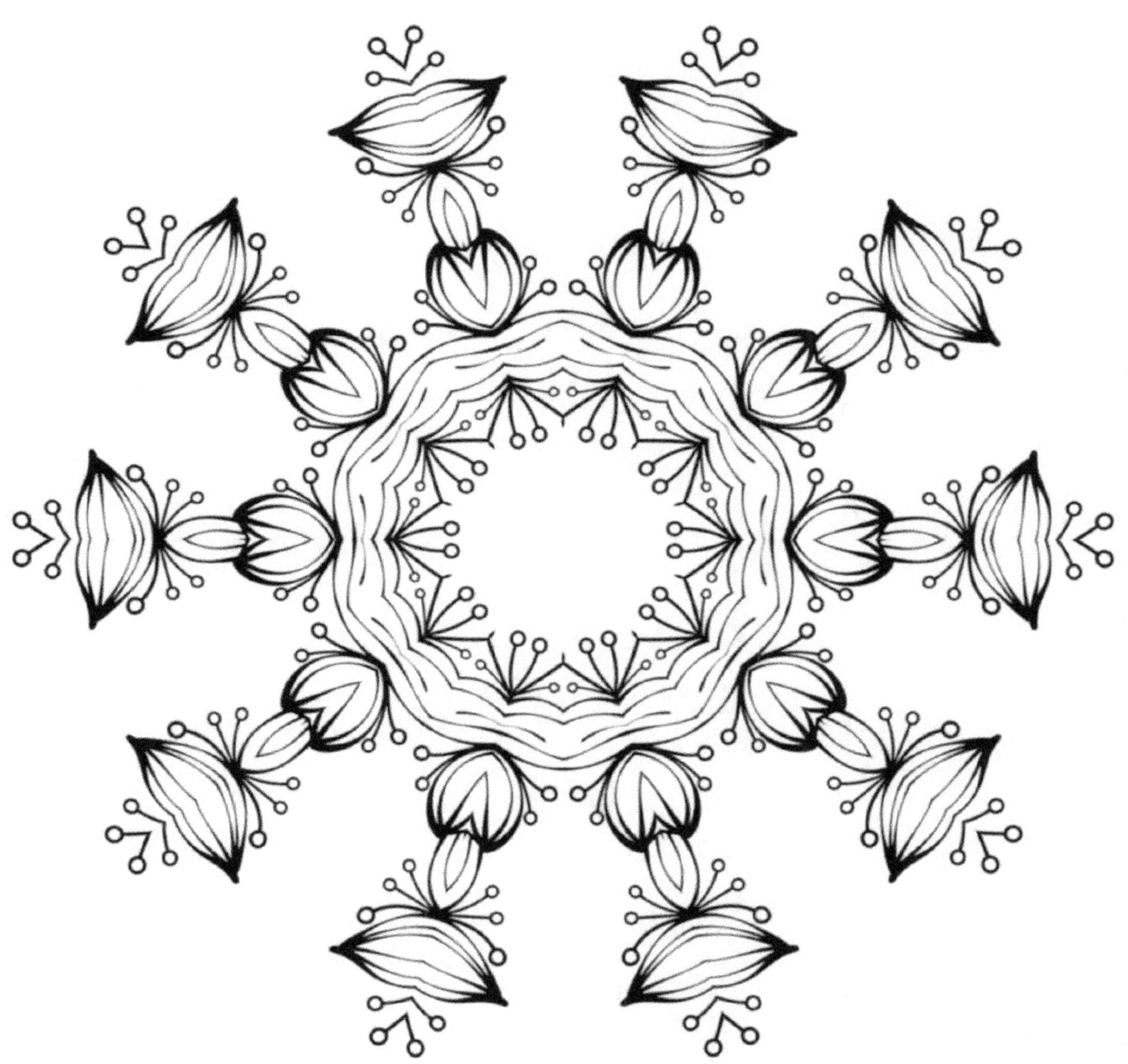

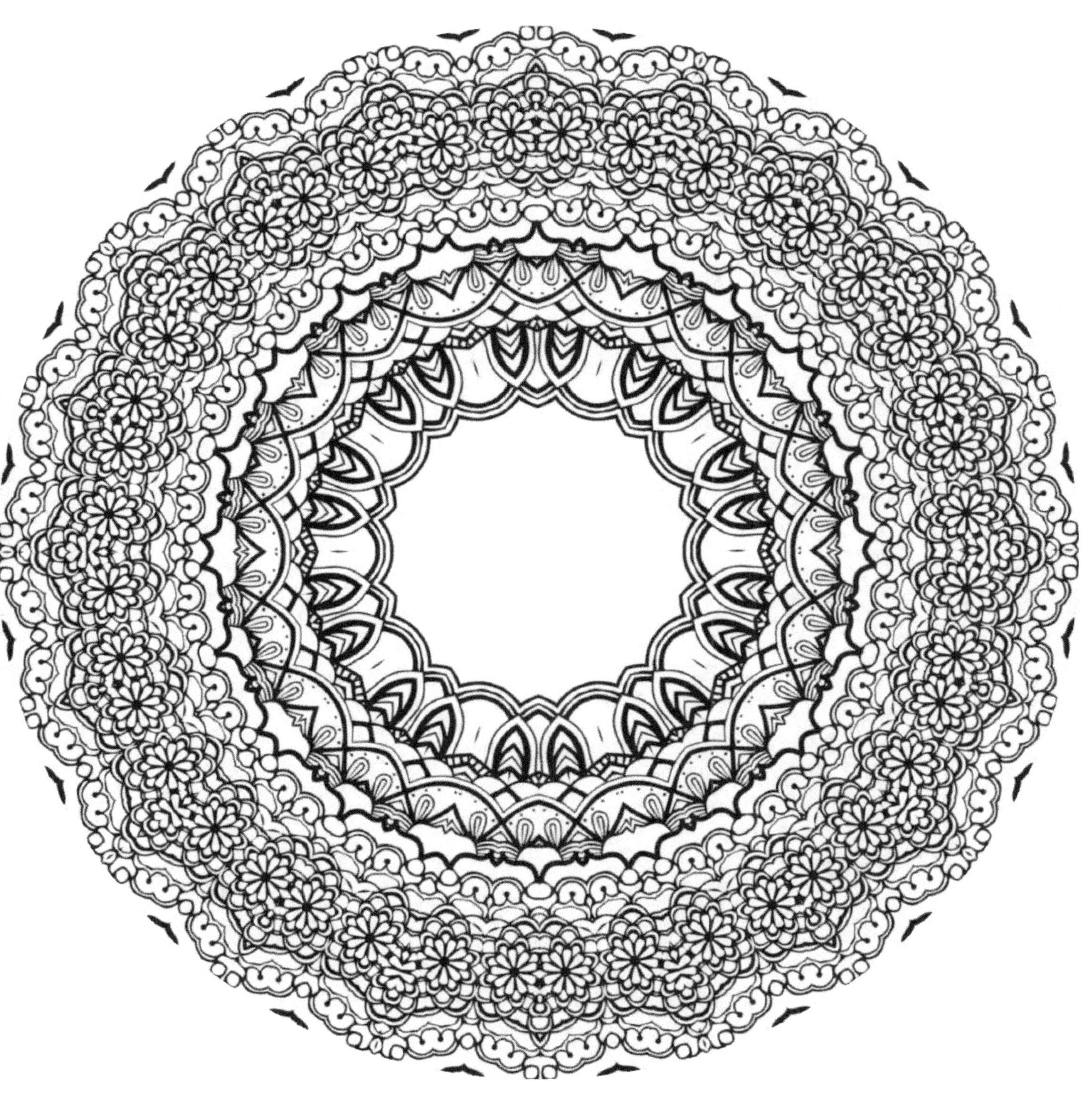

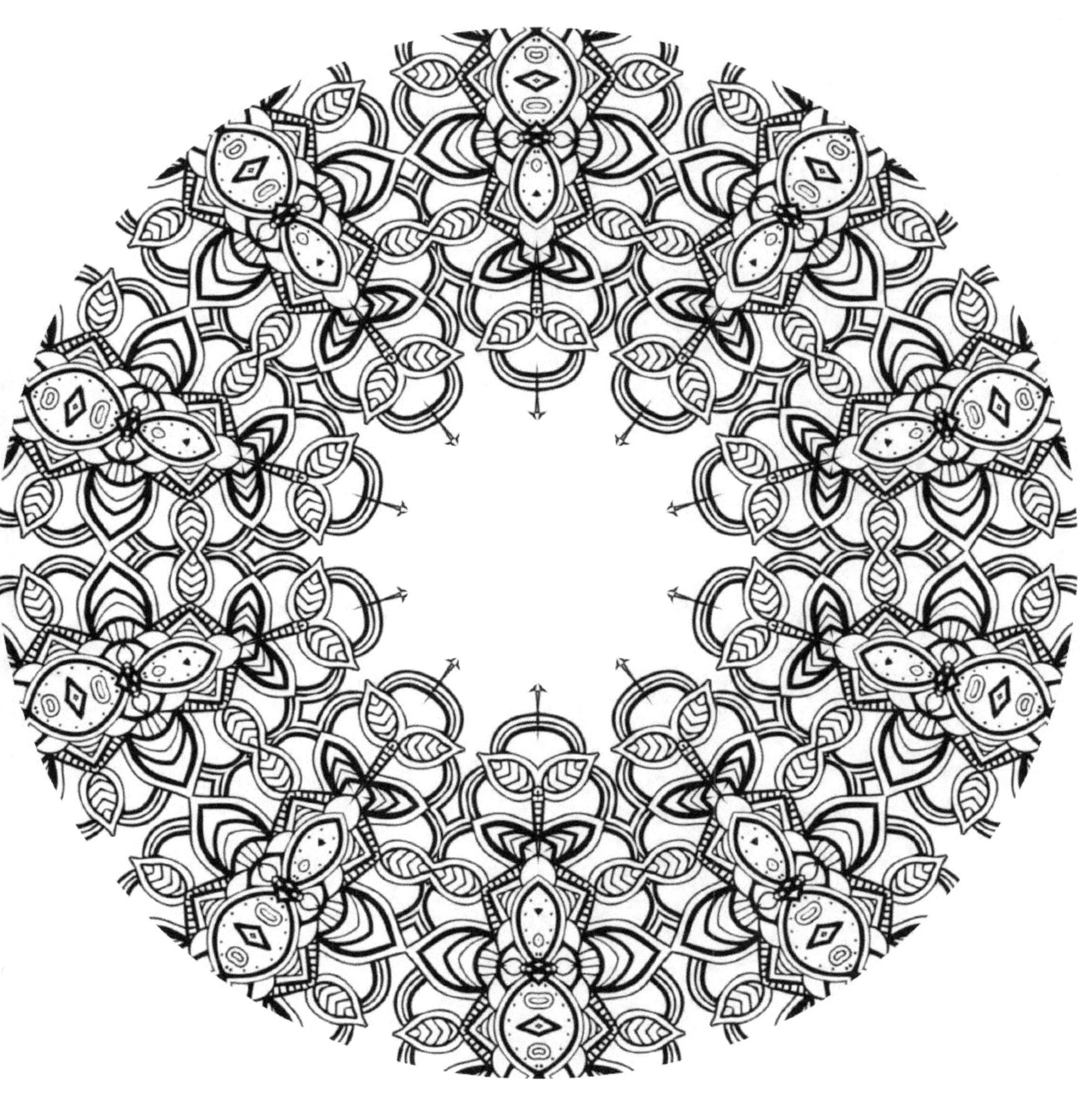

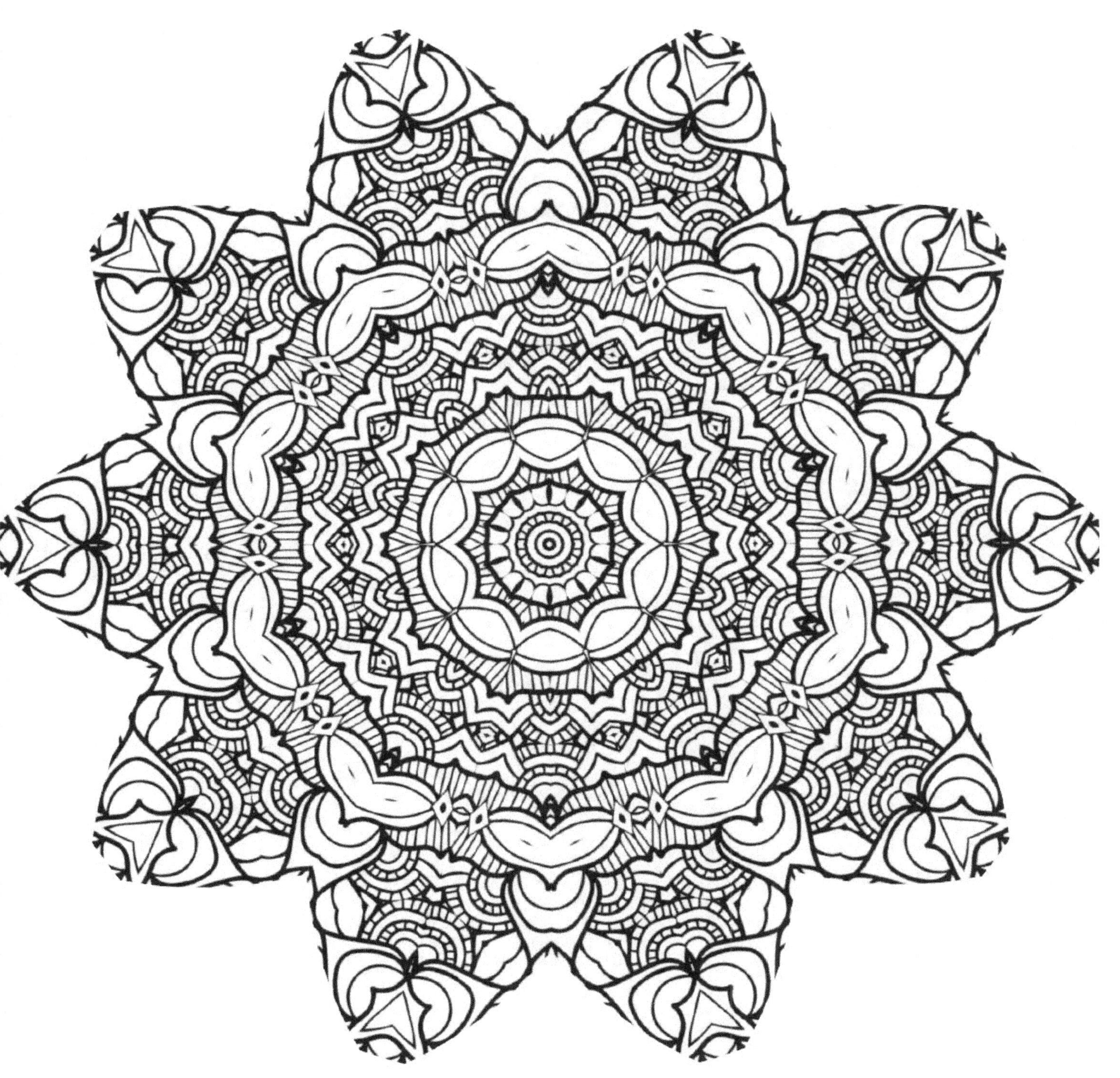

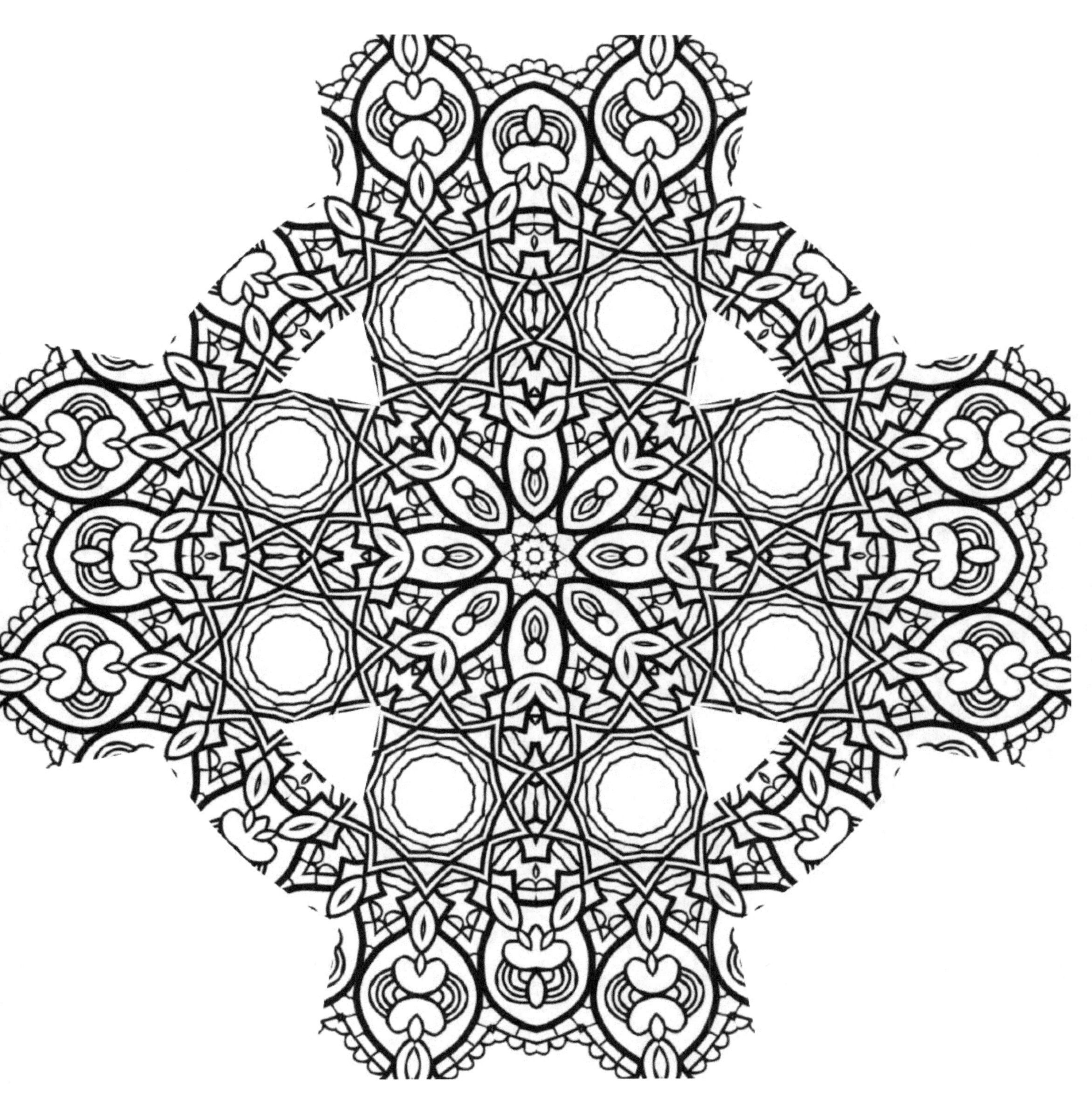

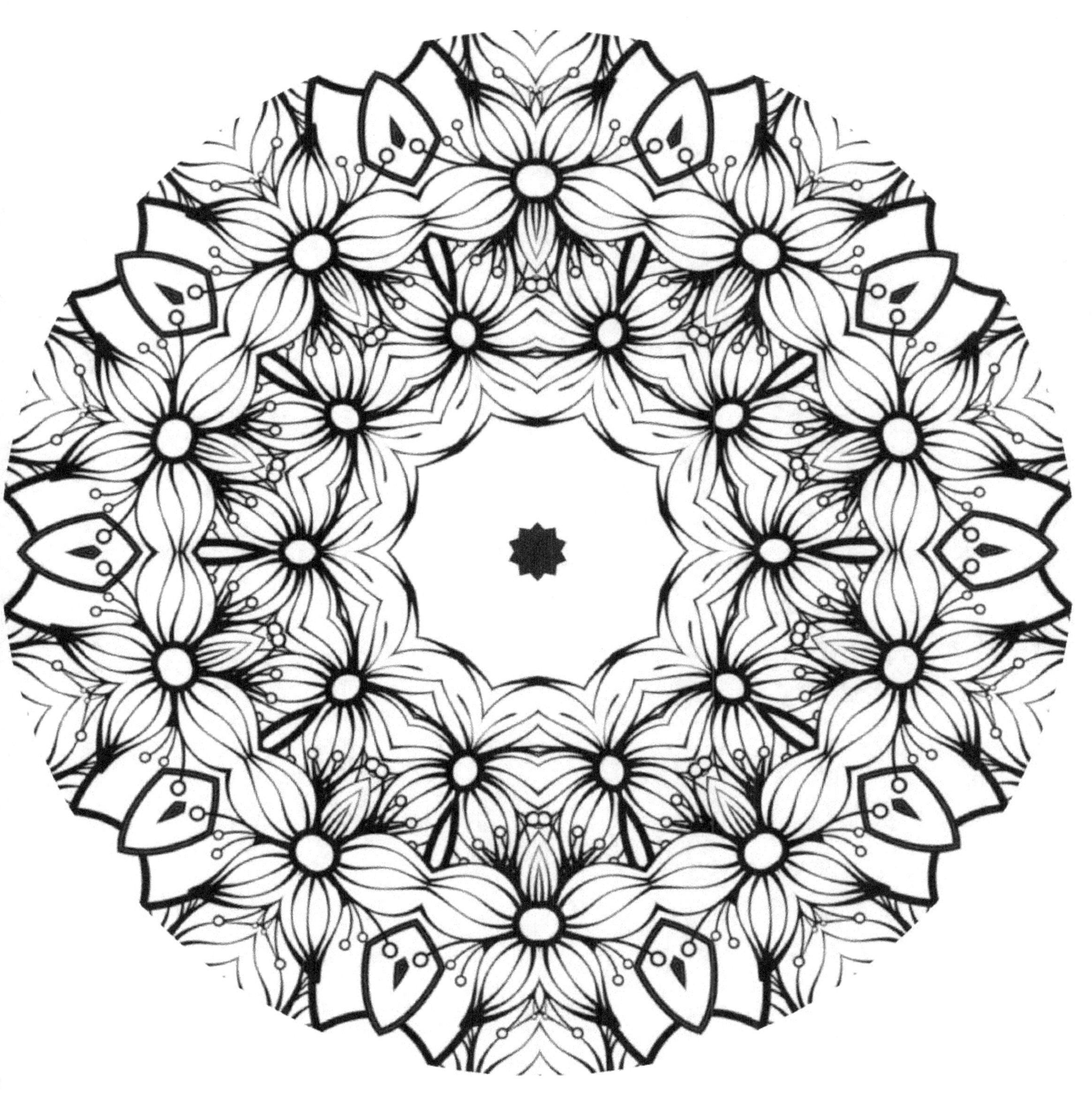

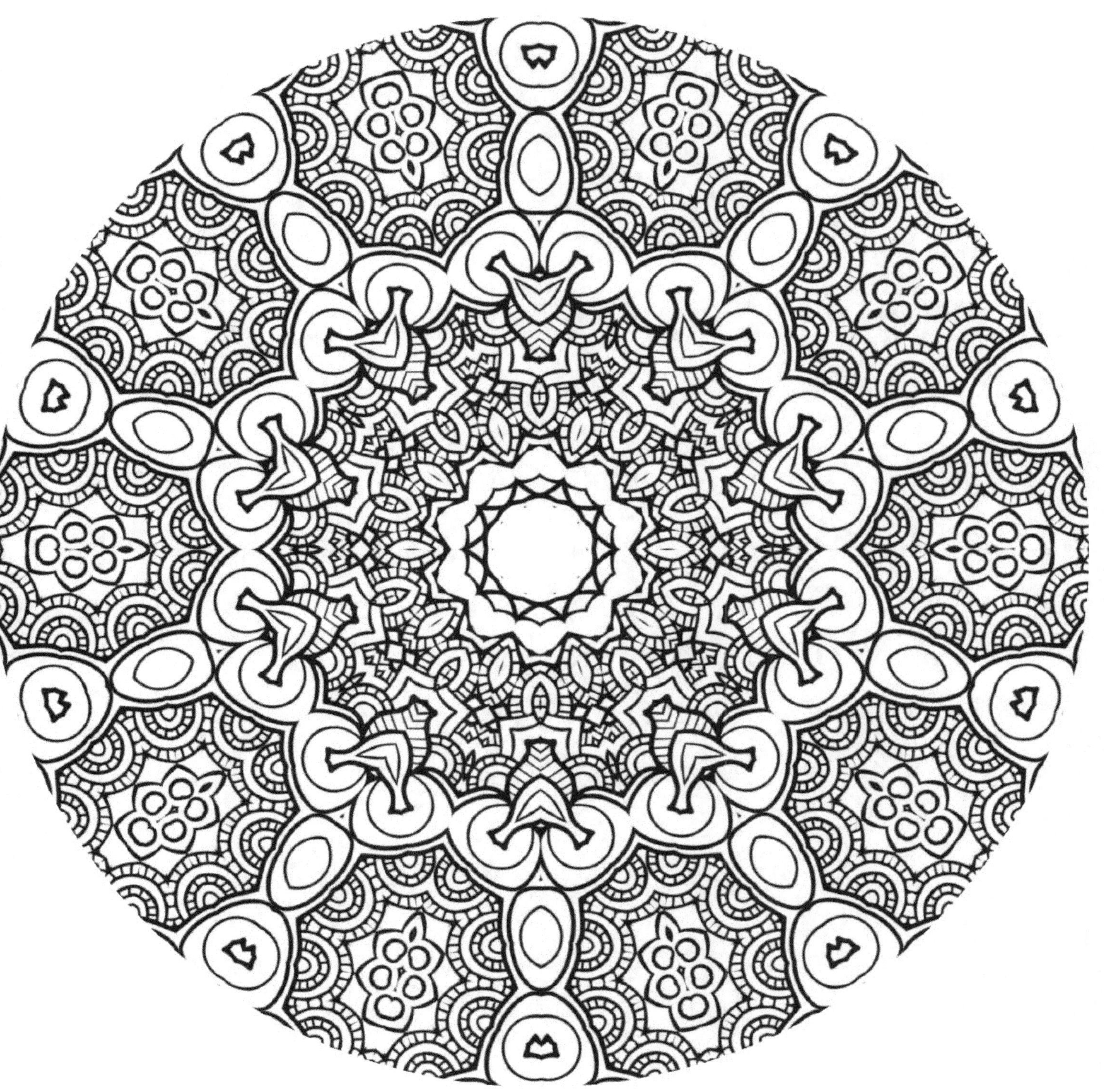

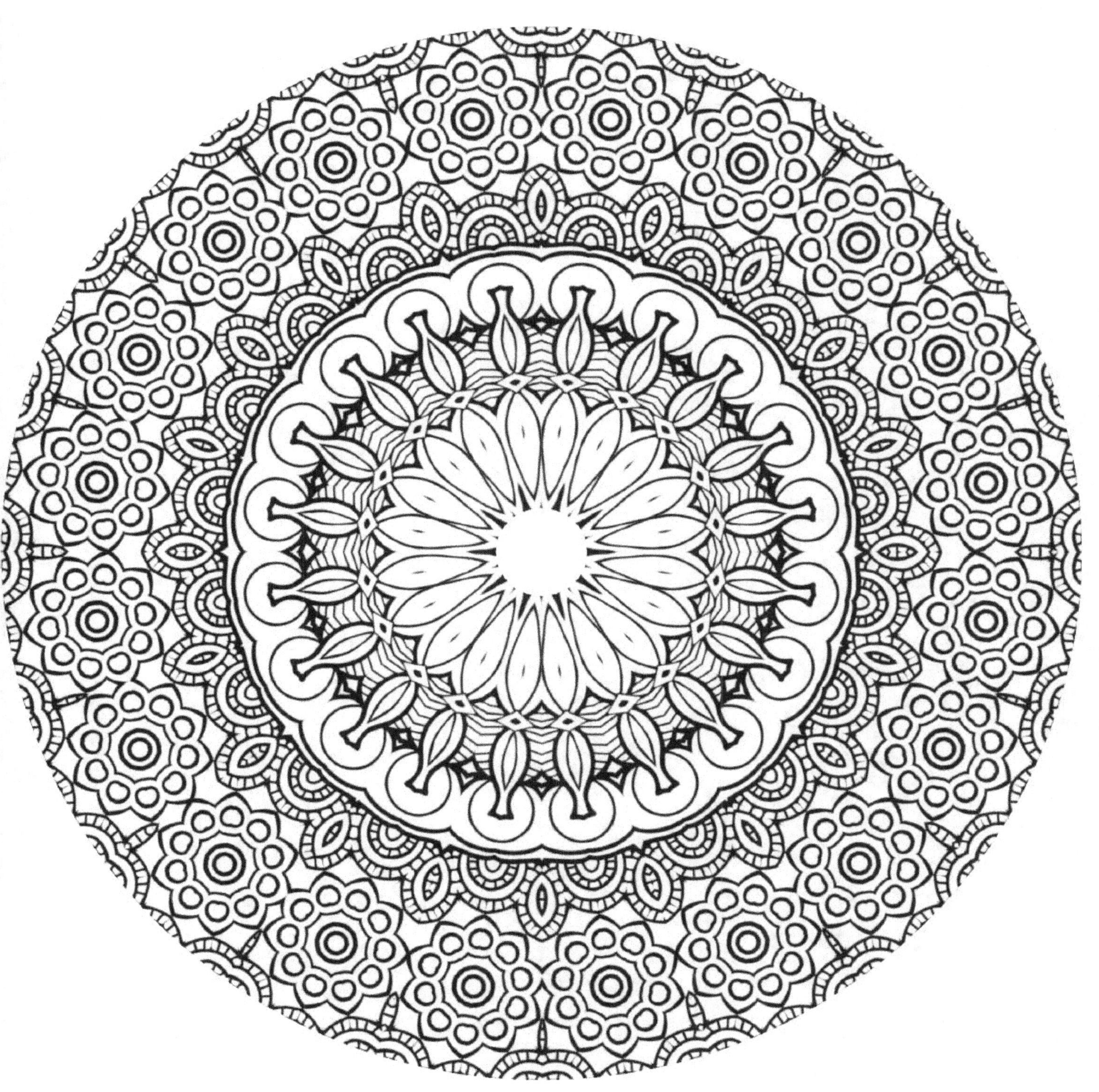

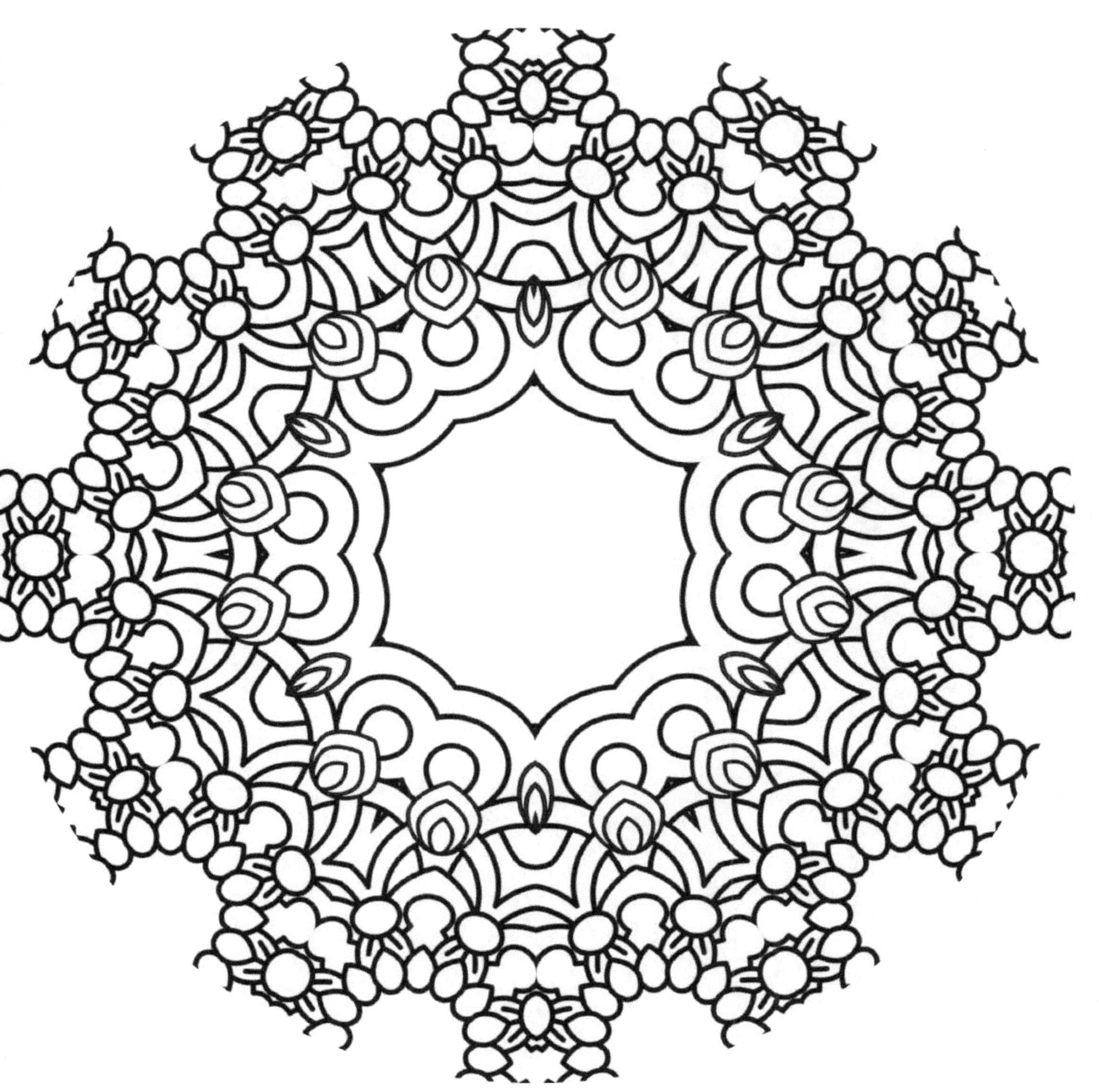

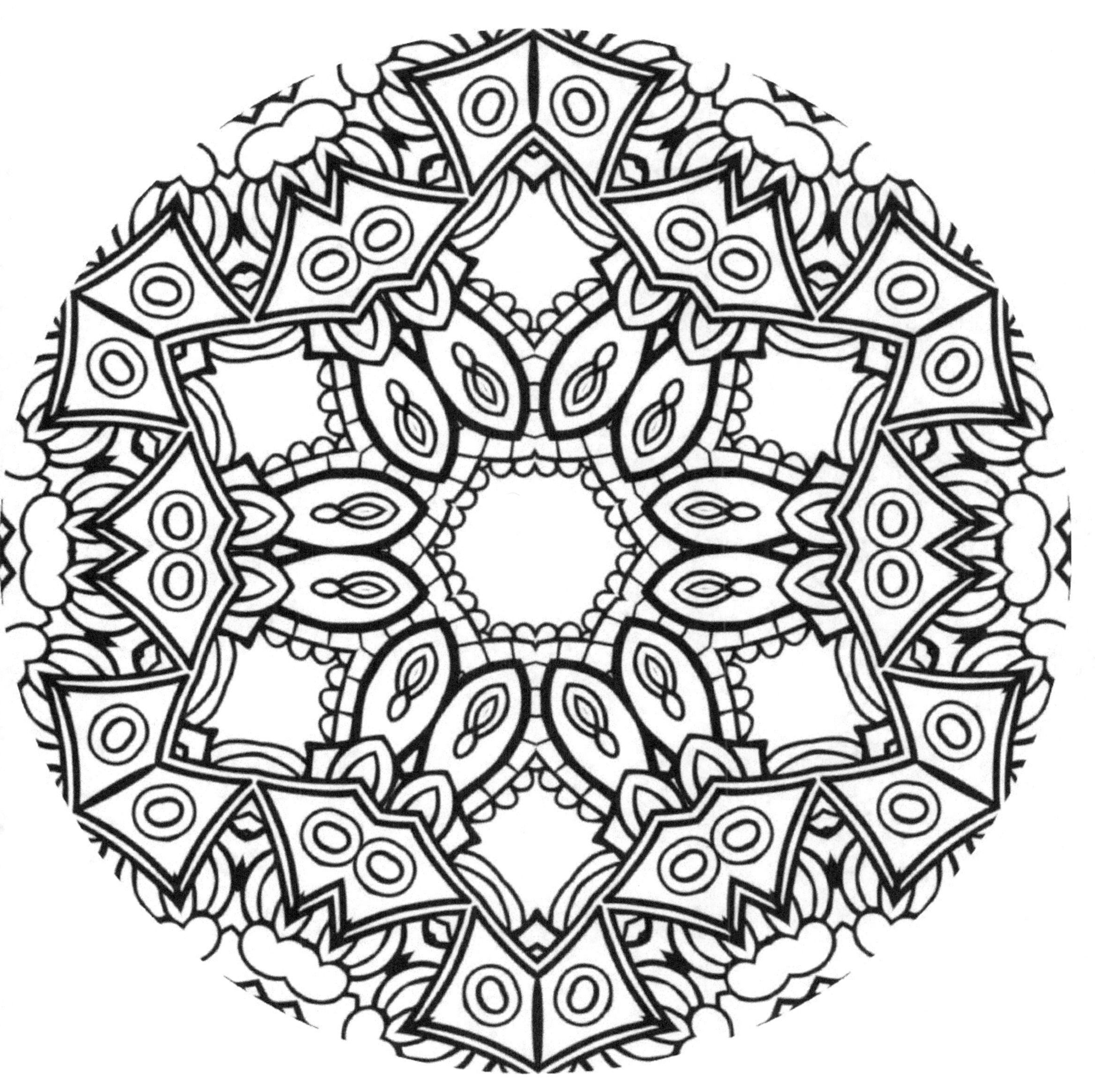

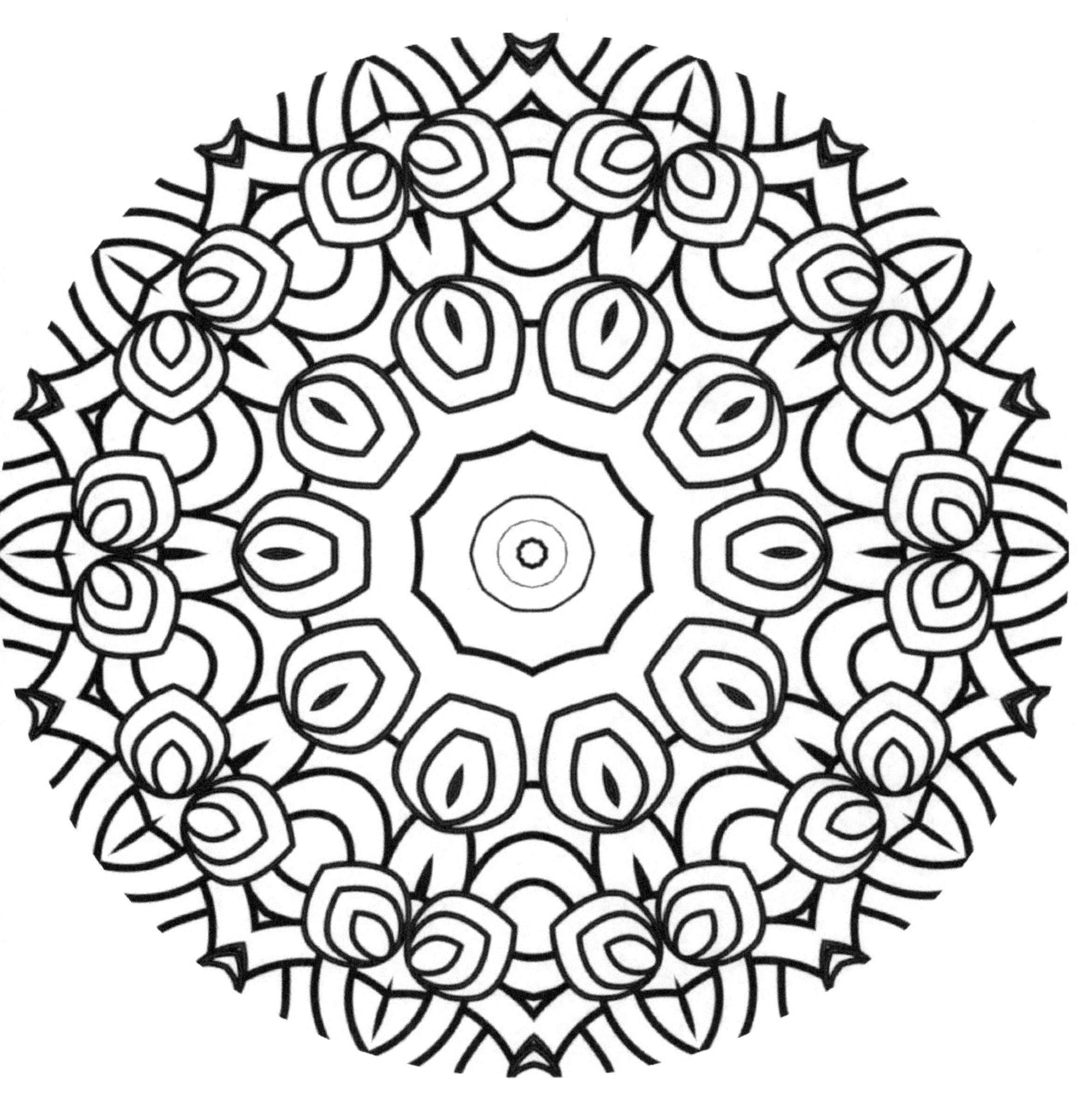